PERSONAL ETHICS AND ORDINARY HEROES

Personal Ethics and Ordinary Heroes: The Social Context of Morality examines what it means to be an authentic hero and provides real-life narratives that underscore the ethical principles guiding decision-making in the justice system and beyond.

This engaging work revolves around a collection of excerpts from students studying ethics and social justice. The essays were responses to an invitation to write about and discuss a hero in their lives who motivated them to be more just, compassionate and morally responsible persons. These essays, collected over several years, portray shared meanings of heroism rooted in themes like sacrifice, perseverance and wisdom. The authors set student narratives in dialogues related to ethics and leadership that are both entertaining and useful for contemporary students and practitioners. This book illustrates the lessons of ethics in criminal and social justice practice and makes them tangible to students. Fostering the benefits of experiential learning, it brings real meaning to students of criminal justice as well as professionals in the criminal justice field and other areas of human and social service practice. It is an essential accompaniment to primary texts used in ethics courses and training seminars.

This book is intended for use in undergraduate classes in applied human sciences and services like criminal justice, criminology, social work and political science. It is particularly well-suited for classes in the areas of ethics, organizations and administration, and leadership. It is also worthwhile reading for the active justice practitioner.

Michael J. DeValve is a dad, spouse, son, author, educator, zemiologist, meditator, mediator and musician. Michael's primary scholarly focus is justice as love. He is interested in police-community conflict resolution and organizational capacity-building, and he is passionate about the arts in the justice classroom. Michael is Assistant Professor in the Department of Criminal Justice at Bridgewater State University.

Michael C. Braswell is Professor Emeritus in the Department of Criminology and Criminal Justice at East Tennessee State University. A former prison psychologist, he earned degrees from the University of Southern Mississippi, University of Georgia, University of West Georgia and Mercer University. He has published in the areas of ethics, counseling, human relations, corrections and law enforcement. His publications also include two novels and three short story collections.

"This book offers a completely different approach to learning about heroes, ethics, and leadership. The reader will be taken on a journey through fable, fiction, and history, but, mostly, using first-person stories shared by students. The reader is invited to think about the meaning of authentic heroism. The authors share with us their students' heroes (the parent, friend, teacher, and others) and deconstruct the elements of heroism through them. This book is supremely timely as we now recognize heroism daily in the healthcare professionals and first responders who risk their lives daily to take care of others. In this pandemic of historic proportions, De-Valve and Braswell give us perspective to distinguish between leaders who are also heroes in their quiet commitment to do their duty, and those who merely posture and pretend to lead."

— *Joycelyn Pollock, Professor, School of Criminal Justice,*
Texas State University

PERSONAL ETHICS AND ORDINARY HEROES

The Social Context of Morality

Michael J. DeValve and Michael C. Braswell

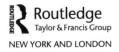

Routledge
Taylor & Francis Group

NEW YORK AND LONDON

First published 2021
by Routledge
52 Vanderbilt Avenue, New York, NY 10017

and by Routledge
2 Park Square, Milton Park, Abingdon, Oxon, OX14 4RN

Routledge is an imprint of the Taylor & Francis Group, an informa business

© 2021 Taylor & Francis

Library of Congress Cataloging-in-Publication Data
A catalog record for this title has been requested

ISBN: 978-0-367-34615-7 (hbk)
ISBN: 978-0-367-34703-1 (pbk)
ISBN: 978-0-429-32725-4 (ebk)

Typeset in Bembo
by codeMantra

Visit the eResources: www.routledge.com/9780367347031

MD: This book is for the heroes of the COVID-19 pandemic. It is for the clinical social workers like Susan Klemme. It is for the local restaurants that *expanded* services to the community like Bucktown (Providence). It is for Stacey Brooker, DeAnthony Brooks, Kyle McElroy, Nate Stevenson and dozens of police and first responders, executives and line staff but leaders all, who I rejoice to count as friends. It is for local newscasters like Logan Wilber who seek to tell beautiful and true stories among the cold, still, frightening ones. It is for health care workers like Katherine Adkinson, Scott Clement and Dr. Aasif Ahmed, and for educators like Shay Davis. These are all personal heroes of mine because they lived their truths unbending to circumstances. Each of them manifests love in the most concrete and distilled fashion. Each is an arm of Avalokiteshvara, a finger on the Hand of God.

I don't know your heroes, but this book is for them, too.

CONTENTS

1

THE NATURE OF HEROES AND HEROISM

When most people think of heroes, their minds often turn to people or characters who do mighty and wondrous things. Heroes are those who "shock and astound and terrify people … and bewitch them" to borrow Anthony Bourdain's imagery (Bourdain, 2018). One might think of characters like Superman – stronger than a locomotive and faster than a speeding bullet. There's Green Lantern, too, wielding a weapon operated by willpower. The Wolverine is an indestructible berserker with a tender heart carefully hidden behind a metal ribcage. And, of course, there's everyone's favorite neighborhood Spider-Man, along with a host of other superheroes. There are heroes found throughout history in religious, political and social movements.

One might just as easily think of people like soldiers, firefighters, physicians, police officers and other criminal justice and public service professionals – real people who risk their own safety in order to protect others. It is easy enough to be deeply moved by their courage and self-sacrifice. Instances that may come to mind include acts of selfless bravery by a soldier saving wounded comrades while under withering fire, the law enforcement officer who runs toward an active shooter while others flee for their lives or the firefighter who bolts into a building consumed by flames at the sound of panicked screams. Such heroism deserves our respect and heartfelt gratitude.

Still, the questions remain: is a hero only one who displays superhuman skills or who acts in an extraordinary moment, putting him- or herself in harm's way to save another? Is there more to being a hero than what Superman can teach us? Just what does it mean to be a hero in the fullest sense?

Soldiers, police officers and others can be heroes, of course, but can more ordinary persons also fulfill that role and purpose? More than that, we might find that the circle of people who we could call "hero" is rather larger than we might have assumed. Can kind, committed and compassionate people who don't wear capes or uniforms, but who enrich and save lives through the long haul of life's journey, also be considered genuine heroes?

The purpose of this book is to explore just what it means to be a hero. It is not mere academic rumination or a contemplation of theory. It is a thought exercise, yes, but it is also deeply experiential in nature. What does it feel like to risk oneself in the moment or over the course of one's life to help someone else? What does it feel like to be on the receiving end, to experience the benefits, short- and long-term, of someone else's heroic acts? In fact, the raw material for this book comes from students themselves. Students in ethics courses taught by one of the authors were asked to describe a specific hero in their lives, someone who helped them in a profound and life-changing way. What they said was revealing, wise and often deeply moving. Their reflection on the real heroes in their lives offers important reminders about what heroism really looks like, and that "ordinary heroes" are *anything* but ordinary. It is our privilege to share with you what they said and the wisdom it offers each of us in choosing which path we will embrace – hero, villain or victim – on our life's journey.

At the conclusion of our exploration into what it means to act in a moral and compassionate way, to be a hero large or small, we will try to put to use all we have learned in our pursuit of becoming more just and socially conscious persons.

Who Jumps out of a Perfectly Good Plane?

A paratrooper's job is an extraordinary one, to say the very least. In the early hours of June 6, 1944, Dick Winters and thousands of his fellow paratroopers leapt from planes into damp darkness above occupied France. Their aim was to pave the way for the masses of soldiers and armor making their way inland from Normandy. Seizing and holding bridges and key road junctures as well as sowing confusion were their aims; little more than small arms and grit were their only tools. They faced a capable but varied enemy, ranging from half-trained conscripts to crack German panzer units blooded in the fighting on the brutal Russian front.

By the end of the war E Company, 506th Regiment (called "Easy Company"), now made legend by Stephen Ambrose's books and the TV series *Band of Brothers*, saw combat not only in Normandy but also in Holland, Belgium and Germany. They fought as part of Operation Market Garden near Nuenen, held part of the front line at a place called "The Island," stood at Bastogne against Hitler's last-ditch offensive and celebrated V-E Day occupying Hitler's private retreat at Berchtesgaden. Dick Winters showed himself to be an excellent soldier and tactician; he was promoted to the rank of major and made battalion commander. His clear leadership, his command of tactics and situation and his unfailing courage certainly saved the lives of many under his command. The men of Easy Company, heroes all, did exceptionally brave things, and yet they turned to Dick Winters, seeing him as *their* leader, *their* hero.

Both of us have tended a keen interest in World War II. It is an interest like that had by many who grew up in our generations, one that does not grow out of a sanguine and unwholesome interest in the bloody and extreme nature of battle, or an interest resulting from contemplating the question of mettle, whether we ourselves might survive and stay the course in the crucible of combat. Rather, it is an interest in the lessons taught by total conflict on such a vast and dehumanizing scale for those who seek peaceful and humanizing solutions to vexing human problems. Both of us know people who fought and contributed in extraordinary ways to freedom's cause, often sacrificing life and limb and heart to that purpose. So let us tell you another story.

A very dear family friend of one of us recently entered a nursing home at the tender age of 94. Until his retirement now several decades ago, William "Stanley" McMillan taught music in a small school district in Upstate New York. Though he was the child of Canadian immigrants, when World War II began for inhabitants of the New World, he did not hesitate to assume duty in the American armed forces. Rather than wallow in trenches, he thought, he would enlist in the U.S. Navy. There being little place for French horn players in naval combat, he was directed to put his ears to work as a sonar technician. He made several trips back and forth between the United States and Londonderry, England, at the post of a sonarman on the USS *Bates,* a destroyer escort. His vessel was redirected from transport escort duty to provide support for Rangers landing on Iles St. Marcouf, a small fortified island outcropping that posed a dangerous flanking threat to the Overlord landing operation. The Rangers found no enemy soldiers there, only mines and booby traps. Due to the need to care for wounded, evacuation took longer than anticipated, and daybreak revealed their location to German shore-based artillery. They watched as shells steadily walked their way toward their ship. As morning fog lifted, though, the vast Overlord armada came into view and the Germans, now realizing the scale of their danger, redirected their fire.

After Overlord, Stan was promoted and stationed in Key West to train sonar technicians, and the *Bates* was sent to the Pacific. Not quite a year later the *Bates* was patrolling south of Iwo Jima when it was struck by three kamikazes, one of which hit the bridge at his former duty station.

No, Stan did not leap from a plane, knife in his teeth or charge up the beach on D-Day. That was not what was asked of him. And it turns out that what was asked of him or anyone really matters when it comes to how we understand heroes. The roles we assume are not always worthy of the limelight, but that doesn't diminish their importance. Stan the musician-turned-sonarman, along with each of his shipmates, is a hero. More precisely, as Stan has become some-one very dear over the years, he is *my* hero. And that, among all the things we will think about here, might well be the most important thing of all.

Well, if we can agree to this much so far, then perhaps our main point is not so unwelcome: there are *many kinds* of heroes. Where the idea of heroism becomes really interesting, and re-ally important for how we live our lives today, is in understanding what kinds of things make someone a hero.

Our first step in the process is to trace something of a brief sampling of heroes throughout history as a way to help us think a little more clearly about heroes and heroism. Thinking clearly and broadly about what constitutes heroes is just what the students did in when asked about their heroes. The complexity of heroism, as the students came to understand, provides us with insights that bear repeating, perhaps particularly so in today's world.

Through our contemplation of the nature of heroes and heroism in the second chapter, we will consider ideas about heroism, heroes portrayed in literature and stories, as well as examples of real people who lived and made sacrifices for what they perceived as a greater purpose. These heroes will be individuals who acted or represented a kind of heroism at historic turning points in both small and big ways. To understand these heroes, we will examine them in terms of the meanings that guided them and the choices they made. The chapters that follow will present the heroes offered to us by the students in thematic fashion. The final chapter will tie all of the themes together and offer something of an avatar of the hero as we understand her or him today.

But hold the phone. Are heroes *of* the moment, or do they *make* the moment? Or could both elements be at play? Are heroes those who see the conditions around them realize what must be done and then rise to the occasion or are heroes those who make opportunities come into being by their thought and action? You might be thinking of the harrowing story of one or another Medal of Honor recipient, someone who saw his comrades in danger, realized the shape of the moment, saw what had to be done and simply did it. Fair enough. But again, is that all there is to the story of heroism? If you say yes, the stories told to us which we will review later in the book might catch you off guard. The scope and nature of heroism is larger and deeper than we might think.

Of course, there's no reason to assume that the "of-the-moment-versus-make-the-moment" choice is an either-or affair: it might well be the case that we can examine heroism merely *in* the moment. Heroes may do either respond to the situation or change their conditions or both. What might be really helpful, then, is to think about how heroes operate in the moment. To the greatest extent possible we should consider their thinking and their action *in context*.

Let us turn, then, without further ado, to our contemplation of heroes and heroism. It is our earnest hope that our time together here will constitute more than food for thought or fodder for an exam or essay; thought about heroes is thought about what we value, who we are and perhaps what is more, who we seek to be.

Questions

1   What are some differences between superheroes like the ones portrayed in movies and ordinary heroes that live around us?
2   What are the different kinds of heroes you have observed or read about?
3   Are heroes "of the moment" or do they "make the moment?" Can both be true, where context and a hero's response to a given circumstance is required?

Reference

Bourdain, A. (2018). The Balvenie honors Anthony Bourdain. YouTube video, September 17, 2018. Accessed September 19, 2018, 2:07am from https://www.youtube.com/watch?v=Iz-5HGDx2k0, https://youtu.be/lz-5HGDx2k0

2

A SAMPLING OF HEROES IN HISTORY

There is an old Basque saying: "we are because we were." The stories we tell, factual or fictional, hold prized ideas like rare gems, ideas prized by those living long before us, offering rich insights into the meaning of their lives. Over time ideas stack upon ideas like sediment. Some get worn away by the human equivalent of erosion, whereas others remain, becoming more polished and valuable over time. Proven sturdy through their durability and refinement, these ideas constitute a considerable part of our cultural heritage in the world we live in today. So it is with heroism. Let us turn, then, to a few examples of heroes in history and their moments of decision.

The Greek Hero in Story

The literature of ancient Greece is a rich source of heroes and ideas about heroism, but here we have space only for a very brief conversation. Instead of a review of all of it, we will consider just two characters from Greek story, both of whom may well already be familiar to you. Both men are ... well, men, and both are soldiers' soldiers. Both of them are portrayed in the *Iliad* of Homer, and both fight against Troy. What will become clear from our comparison of these two characters is that although the idea of what a hero looked like was already broader than merely "the good guy," the idea of what a hero was in ancient Greek thought was definitely more limited than the idea of what a hero is today.

In spite of popular legends and movies like *Troy,* Finley and colleagues make a rather convincing argument against the idea of a flotilla of Achaeans coming from the Greek mainland to recover the dignity of a jilted king (Finley, Caskey, Kirk, & Page, 1964). Far more believable would be the possibility of overland raids from the *east*. It seems possible that some Achaeans might have numbered among the marauders who attacked Troy from the east, but their presence there would be more likely because things were getting rough back home in Greece, and not because they felt it necessary to recover their king's girlfriend or to avenge his wounded pride.

So who are our two heroes, exactly? After all, one might argue the whole *Iliad* is nothing but heroes in swift and violent collision with other heroes. Two stand out, though, at least for our purposes here. The first, of course, is Achilles. By all accounts he is the greatest soldier on the Achaean (Greek) side. He is so fearsome in battle that at one point in the *Iliad*, the fatigued Trojan army scatters in fear when Achilles shows up *unarmed*. Not only is he "of the swift feet," it seems he can almost count on divine intervention on his behalf. For example, legend has it that he was given impenetrable armor made by Hephaestus, god of the forge.

Although Achilles was truly fearsome in battle, he possessed a tragic flaw: prideful anger (Lattimore, 1951). When Patroclus, Achilles' close friend, was mistaken for Achilles and killed by the Trojans (Patroclus was wearing Achilles' armor), Achilles set upon the Trojans in a rage, and killed scores. The *Iliad* does not recount Achilles' death, but according to myth as the Trojan war reached its climax, he was struck by an arrow in the one place where he was vulnerable: his heel.

Our second hero is Ajax the Greater. Ajax the Greater was absolutely *massive*. He was a citadel of a man. Among the Achaeans, he was second only to Achilles. He was just plain mighty. Almost like a modern-day Hulk, the mountain of a man that was Ajax excelled when circumstances were at their most dire. He overcame everything the enemy could hurl at him and simply stood his ground. Well regarded by his fellow soldiers, one could assert without too much difficulty that it was Ajax in fact, and not Achilles, who was the greatest soldier among the Achaeans. Achilles might be fearsome, but Ajax was a soldier's soldier.

We mentioned Achilles' armor earlier. After Achilles was killed, his body was recovered by Ajax and Odysseus. Achilles' invincible armor was a prize indeed, as you can well imagine. The decision was made to give it to the worthiest soldier. Odysseus and Ajax competed for the title and the prize, and Odysseus won … through trickery (Lattimore, 1951). Ajax was so affronted by the loss that, according to myth, he lost his mind, set upon a flock of farm animals and slaughtered them, thinking they were Trojans. When he returned to his senses, he fell upon his own sword in shame.

Achilles was the hero that everyone idolized and *wanted*: handsome, elite, hard-charging and heaven-blessed, even if deeply flawed. What was his reward for his service? Glory, fearsomeness and fierce respect until his own death in battle. Ajax was the hero that everyone *needed*. He stood his ground and single-handedly defended the Achaean camp, preventing the Trojans from pushing the Achaeans back into the sea. What was *his* reward for his willingness to weather whatever tempests were hurled at him? Shame and degradation.

Are these two characters heroes? In the narrowest sense, to the people around them, yes. They risked themselves on the battlefield in search of glory. How they approached their quest for glory differed, mostly because of their circumstances, but both men made choices when confronted with the loss of glory. When Achilles had his concubine taken by Agamemnon, he pouted then left. When Ajax failed to win Achilles' armor, he lost his mind, only to destroy himself in shame when he came to his senses. Achilles was born with the martial equivalent of a silver spoon in his mouth, whereas Ajax had only a broad back and treelike legs. Achilles may have worn a cape, but Ajax wore a dirty battle blouse; Achilles savored the fear of his enemies and the admiration of his allies, but Ajax, even though Homer used the nickname "the godlike" for him, ends his life in shame despite little, if any, fault of his own. Ajax might have had "godlike" as a nickname, but Achilles was the child of a god. In a world where status and privilege matter greatly, this distinction is not a small one, as we well can tell from how things turned out for the two characters.

Both men rose to the challenges put before them until they didn't. We never see either die in the *Iliad*, but myth tells us they do, and not long after. Neither man returns home to family, neither ever has the chance to lift his child into the retiring evening breeze, the chance to know the humble serenity of the hearth, but we might well think of Achilles as being paid in full for services rendered: in life he is honored above all others. Ajax, even if feared, despite being "godlike," remains forever in the shadow of someone else, and in the end exists in Hades as an outcast. In Greek lore, if a herd animal dies unexpectedly, it is said to be Ajax visiting his unending fury on yet another innocent animal. Honored at home in Salamis, commemorated as a soccer team's mascot and lending his name to a cleaning product, such immortality is far from the glimmering countenance left for us of Achilles. Yet it almost seems as if someone who honors service to others might well prefer to be Ajax than Achilles; Achilles knew his life would be short, but he also knew his mother the demiurge; his fate was clear, but so was his inheritance. Ajax gave himself totally to service without any sense of certainty, a thing that might be easy to forget given our vantage in history.

Biblical Heroes: Samson and Paul

The Bible provides a panoramic view of humanity's search to make sense of things. Part history, part myth and part legend, miracles and mayhem abound as tribes sought what they perceived as their God's or gods' blessings, depending on who and what they worshipped. Like we do today, they had their superheroes as well. Who can forget how the young shepherd boy, David, killed the giant of a villain, Goliath, with three shiny stones and a slingshot? Or how Samson killed 1,000 Philistines not with a magical sword like Arthur's Excalibur but with the jawbone of an ass? Of course, all heroes – whether historical, mythical or fictional – have a shadowy side. While as a boy, one could say in the jargon of athletic prowess that David was the undisputed MVP of Israel, his reign as king was another matter. He enjoyed success and many victories, but he also violated the religious values of his people, including having his loyal captain, Uriah, the Hittite, killed so that he could take his wife, Bathsheba, for his own. Perhaps, just as tragic, King David's favorite son, Absalom, led a rebellion against his father for his throne. The old king's grief was palpable when he received news that his beloved son had been slain while fleeing the battlefield. So with them as it is with us in our modern times, on the flip side of the coin that heralded their strengths, their weaknesses lay hidden, waiting to make themselves known. The two heroes we will examine here will be Samson from the Old Testament and Paul from the New Testament.

One might conclude that Samson was the "strongest man in his world." While some heroes become legends after they die, Samson's heroics were on full display in high definition in the here and now of the life he chose to live. Raised to be a Nazarite, one who vowed to not partake of wine or be self-indulgent, he was destined to be self-disciplined and clear-eyed as a judge of Israel was expected to embody. Ironically, Samson instead turned out to be Israel's last judge, given to impulsiveness, gambling, grudge-holding and possessing an appetite for all kinds of women, especially for those from the Philistine tribe. Though a disrupter of the social and religious norms of Israel, handsome, possessing incredible strength and a man of some status, Samson lived life as he pleased with little regard for anyone other than himself. Life was good until it wasn't. The Philistine posse was always hot on his trail at a somewhat safe distance, given that he had killed a thousand of them with nothing more than the jawbone of an ass. As the story goes, what they couldn't achieve militarily, they accomplished with the help of a woman – Delilah who cut off his flowing locks and rendered him helpless before his enemies. We are told that after a long period of suffering and humiliation, Samson repented of a sort and, as a last heroic act, pulled down the pillars of the Philistine temple, killing all in attendance, including himself.

Where Samson's heroics were the result of, perhaps, exceptional genes, privilege, opportunity and a selfish and indulgent attitude, Paul's heroism provided a kind of polar opposite to Samson's life trajectory. He was about the cause he believed in, while for Samson, it was until the very end all about Samson. Before Paul was Paul, when he was known as Saul, he would have more than fit the bill as a Nazarite Judge for Israel. Bright, well educated, self-disciplined and highly regarded by religious leaders of his day, Saul who became Paul was a zealot when it came to protecting Israel's religious traditions. No heretics were safe under his watch. Imprisonment, the lash or stoning to death awaited all who proclaimed beliefs that deviated from the norm, including the "good news" preached and taught by the followers of Jesus of Nazareth. Saul was a dyed-in-the wool "true believer." A true hero to the Jewish religious establishment, he was "Darth Vader" to the followers of Jesus. That was before he had his "come to Jesus" moment.

While traveling to Damascus to hunt down more heretics, he found himself suddenly dumbstruck and blind, hearing a voice that he perceived to be Jesus asking him: "Why do you persecute me?" In relatively short order, Saul the persecutor was transformed into Paul the proclaimer of that for which he had previously arrested and imprisoned people. He was no longer a hero but now a villain – a traitor to the official religious traditions of Israel. Of course, that wasn't the end of his story. Enduring hardships of every ilk and finally death at the hands of the Romans, Paul's heroism was displayed in his dedication and sacrifice in spreading the "good news" to the new religious movement that became Christianity.

Medieval Heroes and Heroism

Medieval heroes had many of the same attributes of ancient and biblical heroes: valor, strength, bravery. Count Roland stood Ajax-like against waves of Saracens until only he remained. He refused to blow his horn to summon Charlemagne, his king, for aid, and he collapsed from his wounds only once the danger to the main Frankish army had passed. In this sense he was just like ancient heroes. Medieval heroes differ from those that came before them primarily in terms of the idea of chivalry. Medieval heroes not only had to be strong and skilled in individual combat but also needed to be loyal to their kings, generous, honest and pious. They should be defenders of the defenseless, of their nation and of the Church.

King Arthur and Sir Galahad

Neither pair of heroes we have met so far – Achilles and Ajax nor Samson and Paul – were totally one-sided characters, like cardboard cut-outs that stand as ads at movie theaters. They were tragic characters with flaws that stemmed from their strengths. Apologists for their inclusion among the constellation of heroes can point to singular qualities but must also be able to "spin" aspects of their lives and personalities that are decidedly less than heroic. As we step forward in time, our next two figures, also a book-end pair, are somewhat even more complicated, and the addition of chivalric ideals is only part of this added complication. King Arthur, one of the most iconic heroic characters from medieval times, was conceived by deception through sexual assault and raised by Merlin, an itinerant mystic. Arthur was destined to be the most beloved king of his people. He faced down many challenges to his rule and to those who trusted him, and it was this trust that guided him, at least according to Tennyson's (2018) poem, throughout his life as king. The other hero we will consider was one of Arthur's most trusted knights. He was pure in beauty and strength and unique among men, embodying the highest ideals of chivalry. He was the son of mighty Lancelot and of the mysterious Fisher King's lovely daughter. And he was quite probably an ass.

According to myth, young Arthur showed himself to be God's anointed king by pulling from a stone a sword no one could budge. His seal of office was his sword, Excalibur, given to him by another mystical figure, the Lady of the Lake. After victories in a few local skirmishes allowed Arthur to begin to consolidate his authority, an emissary was sent to him from the Roman emperor, asking for Arthur's submission and allegiance. Arthur would have none of it. At a time when his rule was not yet fully assured, he chose to stand up to the Roman bully as well as to his local competitors. In both of these campaigns, he prevailed. During his reign, we are told, he established his council of knights, each chosen for his chivalric virtues. These knights were sworn to serve the well-being of Arthur's subjects through the nobility of their character, the edge of their swords and the stoutness of their shields. We are told they sat at a round table so that no one among them could claim to be at the head. Sir Galahad was among those who came to be knights of the Round Table, and what is more, he was one of Arthur's most elite and most trusted soldiers.

Arthur's motivation for creating the Round Table was to establish a force of highly able soldier-servants that would advocate for those who could not advocate for themselves, who would stand up to bullies like Rome and local ruffians. Service to his people was his primary aim, and he understood it to be his divine responsibility to serve his people. He had been chosen by God not merely to be mighty but to be a servant to those who weren't so mighty. Galahad was also gifted with might, beauty and purity, but in the end those attributes did Arthur's people little good. His take on holy duty ended up being an entirely personal one. Galahad's prowess, great though it might have been, worked only to earn him early access to God's side and the glory that went with it in his quest for the Holy Grail. While Galahad and his fellow knights were searching about under rock and log for the Grail, no cities were made safe and no damsels were rescued from distress. At the end of Tennyson's poem, we see Arthur brooding in his great hall, now empty and echoing. A few knights have straggled in from their quests, quests that they now have abandoned. In their pursuit of a holy dream they abdicated their holy duty, Arthur rages; his brave knights "left wrongs" in the lands "to right themselves" (Tennyson, 2018, no page number). Galahad was carried to the bosom of God by the angels but left behind an unholy mess. For Arthur, a king's duty is to his people, regardless of the personal gains he might receive if he were to pursue individual glory, even in service to God. For Arthur, service to his people *was* service to God.

Henry V

Although he was the first king who could both read and write the language of his people, in his heart of hearts Henry V of England was a soldier before all else. He lived an intense – and tragically short – life so common among people in his profession. By reports cold and not very personable, and at times merciless with those who opposed him, he won the hearts of his people nevertheless. In fact, he was so beloved that one of Shakespeare's more well-known history plays is all about him and portrays him as a noble and heroic figure. And so we need to proceed with caution here: the man himself and the tall profile cut by Shakespeare probably differ importantly, to the point that Henry V himself probably does not make good fodder for the contemplation of heroism. Except, well, he beat his national enemy France, and in *extraordinary* fashion at the Battle of Agincourt in the fall of 1415. Shakespeare's story shapes our understanding of Henry V the man much like stories told about Achilles, Arthur, Count Roland and other martial heroes of old shaped our understanding of them, often in sharp contrast to how they probably were in life. Indeed, in the final analysis the Achilles and Arthur we think of today may be more fictional than historical. In the example of Henry V, then, we have a historical person who may not have been all that heroic who, through the story told about him centuries after he lived, appears to us today to be heroic (at the least for his people).

More to the point about heroes being of their time, although he lived in the later middle ages, how we understand him as a hero is in no small measure the result of the narrative about him offered by a Renaissance thinker (Shakespeare). We contemplate Henry V as a bridging figure, then: as a medieval hero memorialized in Renaissance terms.

If one were to judge the young Henry on how he spent his youth, one might be forgiven for assuming his reign would have been lackluster, maybe even disastrous. Raised by Richard II after Henry's father was exiled, it seems he nevertheless spent at least some of his youth in, well, less lofty pursuits. He liked pubs. Upon his ascent to the throne, though, it seems he cleaned up his act. One of his first endeavors as king would lead to his greatest success, as well as his own demise: he deepened the almost perpetual war with France, which we today call the Hundred Years' War. In essence, Henry V felt he had a claim to the throne of France through his father's lineage, and he pressed his claim with force of arms. His strategy was to cross the English Channel at Calais and reduce key regional cities like Harfleur in order to get the French to capitulate. On a dark and dreary late October morning in 1415 near the tiny hamlet of Agincourt, Henry and his fatigued and sickly army absolutely routed the outnumbering (and fresh) French army. Several factors contributed to the rout, including the professionalism of the English soldiers, Henry's tactics and the tactically clumsy exuberance of the French knights. The end result, though, was that Henry had successfully asserted his claim on France; when Henry V died not long later, much of Normandy, Brittany and Burgundy were in English hands.

But here is where things take a darker turn. Even as the battle of Agincourt was concluding and English victory was becoming evident to all, a skirmish behind the lines near the English camp drove Henry to order the slaughter of soldiers and knights taken captive during the fight. Even though the English victory was clear, they were still too few to fight on two sides, he reasoned, or to contend with captives who forcibly vied for their freedom. Now, we need to remember that for a common soldier to take a knight captive in battle was not only a laudable feat of arms, it was also like winning the lottery; the ransom the soldier could demand might well make him independently wealthy. The order was eventually belayed but not before some knights and soldiers were put to the dagger. Putting aside the decidedly barbaric, perfidious, unchivalrous and unheroic nature of Henry's command to kill prisoners of war taken according to long-accepted practice, the order to slaughter prisoners was tantamount to asking his soldiers to tear up winning Powerball lottery tickets. Holding up Henry V as an example of heroism, then, needs to be done with more than a little caution.

And lest we forget, Henry's claims to the title of hero meet with the greatest sympathy among English audiences. The French thought rather less of the man. The possibility that Henry was poisoned by the French has been thrown about and cannot fully be dismissed. The French would have their own unlikely hero in response to Henry and his marauders, too: Joan of Arc.

Renaissance Heroism: Galileo

As we have seen already, some heroes are heroes because of the stories we tell about them and not necessarily because of who they were in life. The ironic thing about Galileo is that although he did indeed live, and did indeed stand for some heroic ideas, his heroism was constructed in part by storytelling and, perhaps, a little misinformation. Of course, the story that made him a hero is also somewhat telling, so instead of comparing two different heroes, we will consider two different stories about the same hero. From our consideration of these two stories, we will seek to learn something not so much about them (or him) per se but about how we think about *who* we think about as heroes.

Poor Galileo: we think of him as he faced the fearsome Inquisition, meekly gesturing to his sky charts of planetary movement, stared down upon by unreasoning and doctrinaire judges. Forced on pain of torture and death to recant his belief in heliocentrism (the idea that the sun is at the center of the solar system, and that the earth is merely one planet among several that orbit it), Galileo represents to many the hero that speaks for reason against a blind, oppressive and misguided authority. It is a contest between unreasoning and blind faith against scientific reason. Galileo, we are told, concedes defeat and so saves his own life, but has the final victory of being absolutely right, and the Catholic Church leadership of the time ends up with egg on their faces for all of history. In this particular battle of science-versus-faith, science eventually wins. As a hero to scientists, Galileo didn't pick a fight, but in schoolyard terms, although he yielded a fight to the bully, the bully got his comeuppance in the end, serving perpetual detention in the principal's office.

Except not so much. You see the actual story isn't anywhere near that simple, and Galileo isn't remotely as resolute, nor was his danger anywhere near so dire or immediate. Galileo has become the very emblem of nobility for those who have suffered for the sake of reason against willful ignorance and prejudice, but that may not be as richly deserved as one might think, and in fact there are some real problems with the idea of Galileo as a hero.

Galileo, it turns out, was not as ardent an advocate of heliocentrism as he is often thought to be, and the Church was not as aligned against him as a thinker as we have been led to believe (Kelly, 2016). Moreover, the whole story about Galileo as a brave scientist speaking truth to ecclesiastic power was created by John William Draper and Andrew Dickson White (e.g., Ball, 2014) to advance their notion of the "Conflict Thesis," the idea that faith and science represented fundamentally irreconcilable positions. To be sure, the Church had little patience for heliocentrism as an idea, but again, given the science of the time, they weren't alone in this. *Most other scientists* also held that geocentrism was the state of knowledge; heliocentrism wasn't merely heresy but also scientific quackery.

It has also been thought that Galileo's powerful enemies sought to undo him, and that his powerful friends kept him from being tortured or killed by the Inquisition. That also may not quite be the case. There were probably folks out to stick it to Galileo, folks happy to let the Church do their dirty work for them, but they were relatively few and were at most responsible for the earlier and more benign efforts of the Church to intervene against Galileo. The collision between Galileo and the Church actually occurred in two somewhat separate events separated by more than thirty years, as opposed to a three-decade effort to silence Galileo. In a nutshell, the case against Galileo for heresy was always thin. In the end, all the Church succeeded in doing was to find him guilty of a "lesser included offense" – strong suspicion of heresy. It seems very clear that Galileo was aware of the chance of torture and death at the hands of the Church. Galileo also probably knew his chances of being tortured were quite small, given his advanced age, given that his friend was the pope and finally that most, if not all, of Galileo's enemies had died well before the second event of Galileo's ecclesiastical trouble.

The conflict between Galileo and the Church may be better understood for our purposes in terms of the nature of human knowledge and how humans have approached knowing and experiencing their world over time. As we are thinking about heroes in this project, we might consider this conflict as being between two different approaches to experts and expertise (e.g., Feyerabend, 1985), and thus who counts as heroes. Feyerabend gives us two views on expertise to consider: the first view takes the position that the insights experts produce should be folded directly into the larger human conversation. The other view argues that any insight produced by an expert needs to be examined in light of other considerations (like philosophical concerns or religious doctrine), and more, those insights should be introduced "only when the aims of the experts agree with those of society" (Feyerabend, 1985: 156) to become an ingredient in human discourse. The first view is rather more appealing to contemporary thinkers like you and us; we certainly don't feel the need to take scientific discoveries like the presence of water on Mars or the existence of gravitational waves and ask some philosophical council or ecclesiastical authority about their thoughts on the findings before announcing them. Plato was one who advocated the second view, and the Medieval Church (for example, in the body of St. Augustine) appreciated his thinking.

The struggle between Galileo and the Church was not as much about science threatening doctrine as much as it was about the need to continue to lens science through other dominant concerns, like religious doctrine, before being dumped into the reservoir of contemporary discourse. People like Galileo are held up as heroes for those who celebrate the independent view of knowing; Plato, Galileo's pope and someone like Bernard Gui of the Inquisition might be celebrated as heroes for those who would want new knowledge to be … processed … before releasing it into the wild.

Of course, from a certain vantage such a lensing is merely a kind of contextualization, a thing we do almost habitually today with all good science. In Galileo's circumstance, though, the context brought by the Church was a form of social control; it would have been difficult for many leaders (particularly ecclesiastical leaders) in Galileo's Europe to envision allowing everyone to be contributing to the body of social discourse in a willy-nilly fashion. That context-based control, they thought, made society possible, and indeed such was a fair assessment; for much of the middle ages, the Church was the primary social institution binding a sickly and calamitous, if creative, Europe together. By Galileo's time, though, the need for the social binding contributed by the Church was not only far less necessary than it had been before; it was also becoming clear that it was soon to be obsolete altogether. The struggle between Galileo and the Church, then, is primarily a growing pain; it is a moment of becoming and realization in the transition of Western culture from infancy into adolescence.

Without seeking to diminish Galileo's memory, we think it is important to remember that although he was a noteworthy hero of science, he was also a human being. And like all human beings, he was not without his flaws. Even if we take Galileo as a hero of science speaking truth to willfully blind Church authorities, we are left with the problem of his decision to spare his own life, again if we presume that his life was indeed in jeopardy. And again, our vantage in history clarifies some things while it distorts others. John Martyr lends his name to a certain rather gruesome but meaningful practice; if we hold him and others to be estimable, even heroic, then perhaps it is fair to ask about Galileo's decision-making regarding his willingness to claim before God and the Church his growing conviction in the correctness of heliocentrism. In the play *Life of Galileo*, Bertolt Brecht portrays Galileo's decision to recant as a result of a simple fear of pain. It seems he acquiesced more than recanted, and this choice actively to save himself, made before an Inquisition that did not necessarily seek his blood, is deeply meaningful. If we *do* decide to judge him for his decisions before the Inquisition, though, we need to be just as willing to ask ourselves if, in his circumstances, we would be willing to give our own lives for our own beliefs.

Heroism in the Age of Enlightenment: Cervantes/Don Quixote

Death seems to have come as something of a relief to Miguel de Cervantes. Today regarded as one of the most lauded authors in Western culture, his life was a nearly endless string of professional disappointments. As a young soldier he enjoyed one of the sunniest moments of his life: he was shot twice in the chest. On his hero's journey home from Italy his ship fell into the clutches of slaving pirates; he and his brother were held for a sizable ransom. After years of captivity and three failed escape attempts, his family was able to raise the money to buy his freedom, fully three years after they were able to secure his brother's. The valor of "The hero of Lepantor" (Hatzfeld, 1947: 322) on the battlefield, though, was sufficient to earn him access to positions of influence upon his return home or so he thought. What civil service positions he was able to wrangle were menial, personally challenging and ultimately ran him afoul with his overlords. Cervantes was perpetually short of cash and seemingly unable to manage his financial responsibilities for the Crown. Success with his writing was almost as difficult to come by. Although an entry he prepared won a poetry contest, his plays and novels were unable to win him much beyond a limited, if sophisticated, readership. Only relatively late in life did he know something of the appreciation his work is due.

The Ingenious Nobleman Sir Don Quixote of La Mancha and *King Lear* appeared within a handful of years of each other, and in both cases it would be fair to ask whether it was indeed madness that their protagonists suffered, or an authentic and poignant brokenness. Or perhaps it was something else altogether, at least for Don Quixote. Alonzo Quixano was a simple country gentleman who fell under the spell of chivalric romance tales, like that of our King Arthur. He decided he would no longer be the man he had been, but that he would become a knight-errant and wander the hinterlands in search of wrongs to right. He set himself to the task of assembling his accoutrement; he had an old and moldering set of armor, complete with a partial helmet, made whole through the creative application of pasteboard and wire. His old flea-bitten nag he renamed Rocinante. The last task was to find for himself a lady to woo, like in the stories. A local farm girl, whom we never meet, and he may have seen only once and at a distance, is chosen: he christens her Dulcinea del Toboso, and with her to hold before himself in all adventures to come, his materiel are prepared. Seeing him as quite surely mad, a local innkeeper who Don Quixote takes to be the lord of a castle, along with prostitutes he takes to be noble ladies, together bestow him his knighthood and send him into the world.

Don Quixote sees the world in his own terms; through the lens of a knight-errant, yes, but not only this. Travelers in carriages are captured maidens in need of rescue, a barber's basin is a magical helm and windmills do the office of giants to be vanquished. He sees the world as it is and yet *also* sees another world, not a separate reality, but as a transcendent, interpenetrating one. He sees not merely a fantasy inspired by sappy novels overlaid atop the muddy mundane, but a world as it might be, where nobility and beauty are more than celebrated – they guide action and shape meaning. At times it is a black-and-white Manichaean world he sees where innocent monks on the road are taken to be kidnappers and are assaulted, but it is worth the effort to forgive him his trespasses. Perhaps it is even more precise to say that instead of seeing a separate reality, he asserts and insists upon a separate reality, one that is at the same time far more beautiful and far more terrible than that of the workaday countryside or of the greedy and misguided city.

He intervenes in circumstances based on his double vision and, in so doing, almost always makes things worse for others and for himself. His squire, Sancho Panza, is a simple fellow, seeing things in very plain terms, but who nevertheless gives himself over to Don Quixote's chivalric narratives, and suffers right along with his master. In important ways, Don Quixote sees beauty where others who see things in a more literal and pedestrian sense fail; the prostitutes that participated in his knighthood were held by Don Quixote as handsome and high-born ladies. His insistence on their beauty is itself beautiful, of course, but not all of his takes on events are as estimable. In some of his adventures he proves to be more brigand than hero, assaulting people he meets on the road, taking *them* to be brigands and doing them real damage.

After several adventures, and repeated and *legendary* drubbings, Don Quixote finally returns home where he falls ill. His friends and servants had worried over him through the entire work; early on they burn his chivalric romance books and even plaster over his study to break the stories' spell on him. At the end, though, they reverse; on his deathbed Don Quixote forswears his chivalric oath, proclaims himself no longer to be Don Quixote but merely Alonzo Quixano the Good, simple country gentleman. His friends, once so intent on rescuing him from his delusions, are now horrified, insist that he is Hidalgo Don Quixote, and that his Dulcinea awaits his knightly service. Don Quixote, Hidalgo De La Mancha, died not in battle and not beguiled by a sworn enemy but in his own cold and strange sickbed, without the comfort of his noble and knightly ethic to give his passing meaning and ease.

Cervantes' aim for the work seems to have been to skewer archaic ideas about chivalry. To bring about his end, Cervantes writes himself into his novel, not as the protagonist, but as a frequently sardonic storyteller and judge of Don Quixote. In this his work has something of the sense of More's *Utopia*. More than a few times one can feel Cervantes' elbow in the reader's ribs. Cervantes seems almost to be pointing with his forehead to his main character and offering the aside, "That cat is nuts." In no way is Don Quixote insane, however, regardless of Cervantes' stated intentions. As is the case with More's critique of the society in which he lived, Cervantes' reader is invited, so it seems, to judge Don Quixote, as More's audience is invited to judge their own society in comparison to that of the Utopians', but the *real* invitation to us is to step aside from the judgment laid on Don Quixote by everyone, including the narrator, and to look instead at *the narrator* as mad or dented.

The irony should not be missed here: Cervantes was ridiculing the chivalric ideas that drove Don Quixote, but he himself may have been something of a Van Helsing in a society of strigoi. The Spain portrayed in the work, and in fairness the Spain of Cervantes, had begun its decline from world domination; the people with whom he lived were clawing at each other for status and wealth, which makes Don Quixote's insistence on chivalric principles like storge (courtly) love, and Cervantes' mockery of them, all that much more elegantly barbarous (e.g., Bloom, 2003). Cervantes' publisher bilked him out of the royalties for *Don Quixote*, offering just one more example of the bloated and incompetent self-importance and acquisitiveness that so commonly defined Cervantes' lived experience. And speaking of cruel irony, Nabokov found *Don Quixote* to be hideously cruel for the use of Don Quixote's double vision as a tool for ridicule. Kunce (1993) reminds us, though, that Nabokov's judgment of Cervantes' masterwork could be even more easily applied to Nabokov's own exploration of violent sexual cruelty in *Lolita*, and so we should take his invectives with more than a grain of salt.

Cervantes concludes, "For me alone was Don Quixote born, and I for him; it was his to act, mine to write; we two together make but one" (Cervantes, 2015, chapter LXXIV, no page number). Both Cervantes and Don Quixote stood above and apart, from but not truly of their worlds, and as such they belonged to each other.

Some Modern Heroes

Abraham Lincoln and Robert E. Lee

It would be difficult indeed to select two more iconic figures from the American conscience, two more galvanic and impelling characters, than these two men. The Great Emancipator and the King of Spades stood at opposite sides of a struggle that today still dictates the contours of American discourse and identity. So much has been written about both men that any treatment of their biographies here would be incomplete to the point of being useless, wasteful. Instead of reviewing their well-known lives and moments, and instead of recapitulating their collision as combatants in another comparison here, we propose something of a break in rhythm.

The two men had limited interactions, and probably never met; at the urging of General Winfield Scott Lincoln offered command of the Federal army to Lee via Francis Blair as secession began to unravel the Union. The decision to confiscate Lee's mansion and estate and to make part of it a cemetery for fallen soldiers was made under Secretary of War Henry Stanton and Quartermaster General Montgomery Meigs. Meigs despised Lee for his decision to join the enemy, and Meigs was certainly not alone in his condemnation, although it does not seem that Lincoln would have joined in such condemnation, even in later years as his rhetoric against the Confederacy stiffened (e.g., Kraemer, 2008).

Rather more interesting, we feel, regarding these two men and arguments about their heroism are their internal struggles, and this mostly because for both men the struggles were quite similar. Both men held (or at least tried to hold) ethical positions that were starkly binary, even simple, in nature. For both men, though, their circumstances did not allow for such a luxury as this. Both men turned their eyes to God, investing their faith in Providence, while neither abandoned themselves to events. Each had a firmly ordered ethical hierarchy and each served that hierarchy to the greatest extent possible, though today we might well take a dim view of their ethical schemas. Lee honored his military duty to the nation and abhorred the idea of secession, but felt his higher duty was to his state, to "his people" (Cook, 1865). Lincoln felt acutely the violence of slavery but saw his higher duty to be the preservation of the Union (e.g., Ross, 2009). Both men felt the war that defined their time and place to be abhorrent but necessary, perhaps even a kind of penance for the sins of each side.

We might, as Ross (2009) does, think about ethical claims in relation to the groupings they create among people. *Universalist* schemas do not allow distinctions among people on the basis of identity and recognize both the capacity for reason and autonomy of, and also the divine spark represented by, each human. In contrast, *particularized* ethical schemas place identity or membership at the center of any ethical analysis; group membership creates obligations, and primary memberships thus create superordinate obligations (Ross, 2009). The former principle is an outgrowth of the Enlightenment; the latter finds its roots in the Judeo-Christian spiritual tradition from which both men, and many of their contemporaries in America, came. Both Lincoln and Lee espoused more particularized ethical schemas, even as they sought to honor the universalist ideas in their shared faith. It is this collision, really, more than any other on a battlefield, that should concern us regarding arguments about their heroism.

Lee and Lincoln identified superordinate values stemming from the identities that mattered most to them but struggled continually to reconcile them with the universalist ideas that gave their faith and their Constitution meaning. Lincoln saw himself first as an American, and that in his role as president his overriding concern was the perpetuation of the Union, even if that meant the continuation of the institution of slavery. Lee prized a more local identity, allegiance to the people of Virginia, above all else. When asked to choose, then, although he thought secession was more than mere error, for him the choice was easy.

Both men found slavery distasteful on universal grounds, though both seem to have been able to subordinate their distaste to other, more particularized ideals. One of Lincoln's appellations is "The Great Emancipator," though his decision to free American slaves came not solely from universalist principles of human dignity and value but at least in part from economic interests (see, e.g., Beveridge's biography of Lincoln, published in 1928). Conversely it seems that at least for a few slaves Lee was an emancipator of a kind as well; he helped to affect the freeing of at least 150 slaves formerly owned by George Washington Parke Custis, Lee's father-in-law (Fortin, 2017). As a slave owner, evidence indicates he had few, if any, personal slaves (Guelzo, 2018) but was part of a large slave-owning estate through his wife. In a now-famous letter to his wife penned in 1856, Lee expressed his feelings regarding slavery, calling it a "moral and political evil" (e.g., Blount, 2003), but continued, arguing that the harm done was greater for whites than for those enslaved, for surely they were better off here than from where they came. In this it is likely that Lincoln and he would have found some measure of agreement. From relatively early on, Lincoln had libertarian sympathies, and held fast to "[t]he proposition that each man should do precisely as he pleases with all which is exclusively his own" and that "[t]he doctrine of self-government is right, absolutely and eternally right" (Ross, 2009: 381). The resolution of the universalist/particularist tension found a resting place for both men in the honoring of the humanity of people of African descent, but not their equality with white people. The humanity of those enslaved was not in question for Lincoln or for Lee, but neither was the equality of the races. Blacks were, for both, humans but not brothers.

Both Lee and Lincoln navigated between a Scylla of spiritual hypocrisy and the Charybdis of economic and political expediency. Both sought a straight course and in this both were frustrated. For both, their faiths offered both guidance and challenge; their circumstances offered both encouragement and frustration. In the end, at least for us, neither leadership of a nation nor generalship of an army bears upon the claims of heroism from apologists for either man. Far more significant are the battles each man won and lost with themselves.

Rosa Parks and Claudette Colvin

A number of more modern heroes come to mind, as well as those already mentioned. Dietrich Bonhoeffer, the Lutheran minister, who stood against the Nazi regime in WWII. Gandhi's nonviolent protest that resulted in India's liberation from colonial rule that inspired Martin Luther King, Jr.'s civil rights movement in the segregated South. There was also Nelson Mandela's perseverance through prison and beyond in ridding South Africa of its oppressive Apartheid. And of course, there are novels like *To Kill a Mockingbird* from which heroes like Atticus Finch emerge. Two more modern heroes we will examine are one who is well known, Rosa Parks, who refused to give up her seat and move to the back of the bus in Montgomery, and Claudette Colvin, the "real" Rosa Parks. Hang tight. We will explain.

One of us had a parental advice-giving moment not long ago. The protestation offered by a daughter is probably more than a little familiar to all parents: "But that's not fair!" The response offered was something like, "No, you're right. Darling, life is not always fair. It is always beautiful, however." Now we know that such advice needs to come with more than a little guidance on its proper use and maintenance, but we stand by the statement. We are both insanely proud of our children, and for very good reasons aside from the obvious ones related to their existence. One daughter stood up to a bully and then successfully mediated the dispute herself; now she and the former bully are friends. Moments like that, when a child does something truly mighty, mightier even than most adults tend to manage, well, that's a singularly beautiful experience. Imagine that parental experience of chest-bowing pride, though, followed by sheer and unadulterated terror to the point that you had to sit up all night with a shotgun in your lap for fear the apple of your eye and source of swelling pride would be dragged out of her bed at night, gang-raped and then lynched.

In the spring of 1955, fully nine months before Rosa Parks' now-famous bus-riding protest, a 15-year-old African-American girl refused to give her seat (in the Black section of the bus) to a white woman as was required. That girl's name is Claudette Colvin, and we bet most people reading this have not heard of her. That's because neither of us had heard of her before a *Drunk History* episode (of all things) made her story known to us. The theme in this section will be heroism heralded and heroism unsung.

It seems that Claudette's story is beginning to be told now, though, more than 60 years after her spontaneous and exceptionally courageous act of defiance. *Exceptionally* courageous you may ask? Indeed so: recall that Claudette was a young Black girl in the South who stood up to a white male bus driver and two white male police officers. Others who had done similar things had ended up brutalized, some hung as well. And her treatment by the officers who took her into custody was anything but respectful. They mocked her body and insulted her with racial epithets, and then threw her in an adult cell in the city jail (Adler, 2009). Her pastor and mother bailed her out; by the time she got home, word had spread through the Black community of her act of defiance. Shoulder to shoulder with pride grew fear for her safety. Neighbors helped Claudette's dad keep watch for Klansmen who sought to teach her and everyone else a lesson.

The local chapter of the NAACP of which she was a member contemplated using her protest and arrest as a moment on which to build a movement, but it was felt that she did not engender respectability sufficiently to cultivate sympathy in the white community (Schwartz, 2009). Nine months later, on the first of December 1955, Rosa Parks, secretary of the Birmingham chapter of the NAACP and a well-known, well-respected (and more lightly complected) member of the community, performed a carefully planned act of defiance identical to Claudette's. Her act of protest gave rise to the Birmingham bus boycott.

Claudette's protest was also not the first challenge to segregation in busing and was not even the first in Alabama. Irene Morgan challenged bus segregation on interstate bus routes (Schwartz, 2009) and won *in 1944*. Almost a year before Claudette's protest, Jo Ann Robinson wrote to protest the humiliation of segregation in busing in Montgomery (Schwartz, 2009). Others protested as well and remain obscure while Rosa Parks (who played a very limited role in future protests and in the larger civil rights movement) became the single symbol of courage in response to violently degrading racist policies. The court challenge that succeeded in ending busing segregation was *Browder v Gayle* (142 F. Supp. at 707); the plaintiffs were Aurelia Browder, Claudette Colvin, Susie McDonald and Mary Louise Smith. Rosa Parks was given the Presidential Medal of Freedom by Bill Clinton in September of 1996. When she died, special legislation was passed to create an exception which made it possible for her to Lie in State before being charitably interred. Claudette retired from a career as a nurse and lives a quiet life in the Bronx.

One other unsung hero is Claudette's teacher, whose name we simply do not know. Claudette had been learning about Sojourner Truth and Harriet Tubman in school right before the incendiary incident. She tells us that she felt their hands on her holding her down when confronted by white authority figures (Adler, 2009). It is an act of bravery to teach about Black history *of any kind* in 1955 Birmingham, Alabama, let alone to teach about the heroism of Truth and Tubman.

It is important to emphasize here that we mean no disrespect to Rosa Parks' memory or act of defiance. What she did was also exceedingly brave, and she serves admirably to highlight the violence of racist policies. Indeed, it was her respectability that made her so perfect for the role she assumed for history. What we must remember, though, is that her bravery was emblematic of the bravery of *many* who stood up to racist policies and culture at considerable risk to life. There was a very real need to manage appearances for leaders of the civil rights movement like Fred Gray, Ralph Abernathy and Martin Luther King, Jr.; great care was necessary to craft the challenge narrative they were to present to the rest of the world. They could not seem to be too militant in their efforts to highlight the violence they faced. We need to be careful not to hold their decision-making in contempt in this regard. We should recognize, though, that the violence of racism perpetuated against them was so profound that it ended up authoring a kind of unintended violence by their own hand against others in the movement through necessitating the diminution of their contribution to the wider effort to confront racism. In the final analysis, though, both Colvin's authentic inspiration and Parks' deliberate action were necessary for the Civil Rights Movement to be effective.

Conclusion

ANDREA: "Unhappy is the land that breeds no hero."
GALILEO: "No, Andrea, unhappy is the land that needs a hero."

Brecht's (1966) point here is that truth should matter above all, even (and maybe especially) before the firing squad. But Galileo hedged his bets and wrote his treatise with more than a little plausible deniability baked in. When the chips were down, it seems possible that his fear of pain was more pressing than his love of truth. Another meaning is to be found here, though, in the space between these two quotes from *Life of Galileo*: although heroes are a resource to be cherished, heroes are the result of need. Heroes become heroes because something is amiss, someone is in peril. Superman would find himself out of a job if humans didn't find themselves getting sideways with each other and with nature on a regular basis; if we didn't need saving all the time, Captain Marvel could go on more fishing vacations and Spider-Man could spend more time with his model train collection. Maybe Batman would learn to play the clarinet.

Of course, the particular shape of need is crucial to contemplate here; we might want a certain kind of hero to show up and save the day, but that isn't always what happens. Most likely when we get a hero to answer the call it is the hero we *need*, not the hero we may *want*. That's because what we may want is not necessarily a result of what we actually need. Consider, for example, Ajax and Achilles. Achilles was the slicker dude of the two by far, but it was Ajax, and not Achilles, who saved the Achaeans from being thrown back into the Aegean. We might also remember Galahad and Arthur: Galahad might be more pious and pretty, but he was also gone. Arthur stayed. Arthur served. We might regard Galahad as an appealing hero, but he wasn't a fraction of the hero Arthur was, if for no other reason than Arthur answered the call to serve. Then there is Paul: imagine the early Christians' surprise to find that Saul, one of the chief authors of their oppression, not only had converted to Christianity but had become a prolific correspondent and teacher! And don't forget Abraham Lincoln. Emancipation was not his chief concern; as we have seen he did not place the universalist principles of his faith and his Constitution first in his ethical ordering of things. Although he authored emancipation, it was not for the reasons we might have hoped. Lest we forget, if he could have preserved the Union by preserving slavery, he would have.

Heroes, we can already well see, are imperfect. They fail. They cling to things that injure them, and in their clinging they lose, just like the rest of us. Samson's strength lived side by side with moral weakness; he failed right up to the point where he didn't (if we take his revenge on the Philistines to be a kind of perverse success). Galileo succeeded in failing to stand firm, and it took some misguided publicists several centuries to turn him into a hero, now often misused. In the end we learn that Arthur's efforts were for naught; his chivalric order later crumbles and his beloved Guinevere runs off with mighty Lancelot. Henry V dies not long after Agincourt, leaving his infant son as king, soon to be defeated in France by Joan of Arc and the Dauphin. Don Quixote disdainfully renounces his knighthood and the chivalric values that had inspired him as he lay dying in his bed alone, surrounded by those who loved him.

We might take all this to mean that there *are* no real heroes, that we build them from spare parts of stories scattered about on the dirty floor of history. Not so. Indeed, quite the opposite is the case. One of the most beautiful things about heroes is that they fail. They are not born heroes but *become* that which they are through a process of not being what they are... until they are what they became. We can see this process at work in several of the examples we have considered so far, like with Samson, Don Quixote, Arthur and Henry V. Don Quixote as a character might not be seen as a hero at all if we view him from the confines of the novel in which he lives and the narrow intentions of the author that created him. It is only with the perspective of time that we see more clearly with a poetic and melancholy joy the nobility of serving a beautiful idea for its own sake, even though doing so is a lost cause. We meet both Arthur and Henry in their youths, at times in their lives when their future stature would be hard to envision. Arthur was not raised in privilege; before he pulled the sword from the stone, he was just a young lad. Henry was born into royal sur-roundings but tended to find the barometric pressure in taverns more to his liking than the rarified atmosphere of the royal court. Neither Arthur nor Henry showed their royal mettle before ascend-ing the throne, but both chose to rise to the occasion of their royal office once they assumed it.

Ahh, choice. Heroes make heroic choices. But we need to be very careful here. If they seek to be revered by others, if they seek the office of hero for the sake of the praise and glory, we might be more hesitant to invest them with the title of hero. That hasn't always been the case, of course. Reward seems to be central to heroic action in the *Iliad*: heroes deserve cool "things" like women, wine, praise and impenetrable armor. Both Ajax and Achilles excelled in their own ways in the claustrophobic model of heroism shaped by single combat, defined by bravery and skill, and conferred through the receiving of earthly rewards. Galahad isn't much different from Achilles, really, save for where his rewards were kept for him. Don Quixote might be the crowning example of the importance of choice-making in hero-making: his entire worldview was itself a grand choice. He chose to insist upon a kind of poignant beauty that no one else could possibly see even if they could at times participate in it. When he chose to abjure his earlier choice, he was choosing to end himself but not merely to die. It would have been only too easy to seek a knight's death in the saddle, serving his Dulcinea. His choice to return to his earlier life was a choice to accept utter oblivion. Choice was critical for both Claudette Colvin and Rosa Parks, but for each we see two very different kinds of choices at work. Claudette Colvin acted from sudden, almost transcendent, inspiration; she said "no" when no such real precedent had existed in any locally relevant way. Her "no" came from inside without warning, but as she indicated her choice was facilitated by Sojourner Truth and Harriet Tubman in the body of Claudette's unnamed teacher. For Rosa Parks, the decision to protest bus segregation was much more deliberate, even if the particular moment for her rebellion had not been chosen in advance. As we have indicated already, both kinds of choice are necessary, both are heroic. Paul, Samson, Arthur, Lincoln and Lee also all had key moments of choice-making that resulted in their being commemorated as heroes by some and branded as enemies by others.

We cannot forget, though, that what a hero seeks to do – the end itself for which she strives through her action and reflection – is a vital component in the determination of hero-ness. As we have already noted, Galahad's pious purity is not real purity; Arthur's dirty fingernails are far more beautiful. Samson's choice to pull down the temple poses something of a challenge for us as it is an act of revenge. Then again, Achilles might well regard it as heroic without the merest hesitation. It does not matter for us, truly, that Don Quixote's giants are windmills. He sought to overlay the beauty in him onto the barren and blooded world around him. It might well matter for us, though, that his nobility evaporated when he ceased to see with the eyes of a poet.

We are inevitably in and of our time; we view instances of action that draw our eye and contemplate them with our own particular hero-colored lens. Today we might judge Achilles or Galahad to be selfish fools, whereas in their times they were tailor-made by their chroniclers to be ideal heroes. For those who honored Achilles, a teenage girl would be about as far from heroic as one could get. As far as we are concerned, Claudette Colvin is among the mightiest heroes on our list so far. From this we should have the realization that the label "hero" tells us at least as much about who uses the word as it does about the person or people upon whom it is used.

We will be returning to and enlarging on these themes as we examine the heroes students described in the chapters that follow. In the last chapter we will bring all things together in an examination of heroes and heroism today.

Questions

1   What are some examples of both attributes and flaws in ancient heroes like Achilles, Sir Galahad and others?

2   How did the struggle between Galileo and the church embody Feyerabend's two views of experts and expertise? In the end, was Galileo a true hero? How would you have responded if you were in his place?

3   Choose a modern hero and identify her or his specific strengths and weaknesses. Imagine that you were placed in the same circumstances and how you might react.

References

Adler, M. (2009). Before Rosa Parks, there was Claudette Colvin. *NPR*, March 15, 2009. Accessed December 1, 2018, 9:28pm from https://www.npr.org/2009/03/15/101719889/before-rosa-parks-there-was-claudette-colvin

Ball, P. (2014). Who are the martyrs of science? *The Guardian*, September 24, 2014. Accessed December 10, 2018, 11:21am from https://www.theguardian.com/science/the-h-word/2014/sep/24/martyrs-science-history-galileo-nazi

Bloom, H. (2003). The knight in the mirror. *The Guardian*, December 13, 2003. Accessed November 19, 2019, 11:17am from https://www.theguardian.com/books/2003/dec/13/classics.miguelcervantes

Blount, R. (2003). *Robert E. Lee: A life*. New York: Viking.

Brecht, B. (1966). *Galileo*. New York: Grove Press.

Browder v Gayle, 142 F. Supp. at 707.

Cervantes, M. (2015). *The ingenious gentleman Don Quixote of La Mancha*. Project Gutenberg (Widger, D., prod). Accessed November 19, 2018, 3:23pm from http://www.gutenberg.org/ebooks/996

Cook, T. (1865). Excerpt from "interview with general Robert E. Lee." *Columbia Daily Phoenix 1*, 45, 1.

Feyerabend, P. (1985). Galileo and the tyranny of truth. In Coyne, G. (ed.). *The Galileo affair: A meeting of faith and science*. Proceedings of the Cracow Conference, 24–27 May 1984. 155–166.

Finley, M., Caskey, J., Kirk, G., & Page, D. (1964). The trojan war. *The Journal of Hellenic Studies 84*, 1–20.

Fortin, J. (2017). What Robert E. Lee wrote to *The Times* about slavery in 1858. *The New York Times*, August 19, 2017, p. A11. Accessed November 27, 2018, 1:12pm from https://www.nytimes.com/2017/08/18/us/robert-e-lee-slaves.html

Guelzo, A. (2018). Robert E. Lee and slavery. *Encyclopedia Virginia*. Accessed November 27, 2018, 1:49pm from https://www.encyclopediavirginia.org/Lee_Robert_E_and_Slavery

Hatzfeld, H. (1947). Thirty years of Cervantes criticism. *Hispania 30*, 3, 321–328.

Kelly, H. (2016). Galileo's non-trial (1616), pre-trial, (1632–1633), and trial (May 10, 1633): A review of procedure, featuring routine violations of the forum of conscience. *Church History 85*, 4, 724–761.

Kraemer, D. (2008). "It may seem strange": Strategic exclusions in Lincoln's second inaugural. *Rhetoric Review 27*, 2, 165–184.

Kunce, C. (1993). "Cruel and crude": Nabokov reading Cervantes. *Cervantes: Bulletin of the Cervantes Society of America 13*, 2, 93–104.

Lattimore, R. (trans.) (1951). *The Iliad of Homer*. Chicago, IL: University of Chicago Press.

Ross, D. (2009). Lincoln and the ethics of emancipation: Universalism, nationalism, exceptionalism. *The Journal of American History 96*, 2, 379–399.

Schwartz, B. (2009). Collective forgetting and the symbolic power of oneness: The strange apotheosis of Rosa Parks. *Social Psychology Quarterly 72*, 2, 123–142.

Tennyson, A. (2018). *The holy grail*. The Camelot Project. Accessed December 3, 2018, 4:23pm from http://d.lib.rochester.edu/camelot/text/tennyson-the-holy-grail

3
PERSONAL ETHICS, MORAL PHILOSOPHY AND LEADERSHIP

Some people find theory boring. We get it: abstract conversations about important things like justice, service or other government activity can almost seem to be a waste of precious time. In graduate school one of the authors and a few of his grad school buddies broke the monotony of study by practicing Aikido a few times a week at a local dojo. Aikido is considered a "gentle" martial art. Practitioners learn to neutralize an attack with just the right amount of force placed in just the right places in order to deflect and ultimately subdue the attacker. The sensei (teacher) was exceedingly generous with his time but emphasized his generosity was purposeful. Invariably he would begin class talking about why aikido movement works the way it does. He spoke often in terms of breath, circles and the hara (a person's physical center of gravity), and that Aikido is deeply rooted in and guided by theoretical concerns. He drummed into us the importance of both precision of movement and repetition, as well as the reasoning behind every subtle movement. All of this, the theory, the precision and the repetition came in handy for at least one of us. One of my friends was sitting in his car with his family when a person approached him and asked for change. The person became agitated and grabbed his arm. Without thinking, my friend subdued the individual through the driver's side window while sitting in the driver's seat. The defense he used was not a thing practiced in any aikido class that we took and yet he executed the move flawlessly and effectively without thinking. In the end, no one was hurt, not even the aggressor.

Theory is not an exercise in futility. It is not just "academic." Indeed, theory is *eminently and inescapably practical*. Theory is the accumulated wisdom of people who have lived before us reflecting somewhat formally on experience. Done properly, like the mythical Janus, theory looks two ways. The contemplation of past experiences prepares us at a foundational level for challenges we may confront in the present and in the future. Often, we hear about how the workplace our students will experience will contain industries and activities that do not yet exist. There is great pressure on teachers and educational institutions to cultivate people who are ready for the workforce of the future. No doubt, technical preparedness will aid students in those yet-to-exist jobs, but theory is still the most able and most practical guide to the future. Used properly, theory does not wed us to a technical template for tomorrow but instead arms us with critical thinking skills that enable our adaptation to unforeseen circumstances and outcomes. Mastering ideas can help us more effectively navigate life's many uncertainties.

What we will do in this chapter, then, is to review briefly two different bodies of theory often associated with heroes and heroism. The first of these theoretical perspectives or bodies is normative ethics, or formal thinking about proper conduct in relation to "the good." Often normative ethical theory operates according to general principles that, when applied, speak to what should be done in a given situation, or at least what a person should think about when deciding on a course of action or evaluating the action of others. These theories often indicate how and what should be valued (e.g., virtue, the quality of lives, "happiness,") or the nature of duty. The second theoretical body we will think about and explore deals with leadership. Leadership theories tend to work more like ideal statements about what works (and what does not) in situations where leadership is needed, often within organizations. These two theoretical bodies will be presented separately and then interwoven in the concluding section of the chapter. Our pairing of theories is entirely our own; at the end of the chapter you will be invited to make your own pairings.

It is crucial for us to reemphasize something before we get too far afield, though. Heroism is not necessarily related to either normative ethical principles or leadership. In point of fact, we should be *very* careful about confusing heroism, leadership and ethics, or even assuming that these three discourses are necessarily overlapping to any great degree. Heroes are not necessarily leaders in a traditional sense, and neither are they necessarily beholden to any ethical system's claims regarding duty, value or action. As we shall see in our examination of real-life heroes in later chapters, a hero often transcends and traverses ethical arguments or leadership roles in the act of becoming a hero. In fact, we might well come to feel that most ordinary heroes are extraordinarily ethical and caring and even something above and beyond what a typically good leader is. We will discuss normative ethics and leadership in the context of heroism in order to create something of a figure–and–ground examination of heroism, which we feel will be useful in the consideration of the examples which will make up much of what follows.

Normative Ethics

Parenthood can be challenging and, at times, even terrifying. It is many things as well, of course: exhilarating, fulfilling, edifying, rewarding, even healing. We are both parents and profoundly grateful for our children (most of the time). The moment when one's child is born simply defies description. One's life changes unalterably from the first moment containing the tiniest hands of one's newborn. It suddenly makes perfect sense how hands so small could carry your heart, could enfold the world. But in this moment of joy and gratitude, a new kind of grave concern rises in tandem. Sure, there is a fear of loss; that something so precious could also be so fragile. Yet, there is another somewhat more insidious and creeping fear: will she or he lead a *good and meaningful* life? Will she or he be *fulfilled*? Am I up to the challenge of preparing her or him to *live well*?

Although most adequately described as scavengers descended from scavengers, we have nonetheless managed to relocate our species from somewhere in the middle of the food chain to being the most capable and most destructive species on the planet. Our power can be hard to feel, though, when we bob like driftwood in the roiling surf. Perhaps that powerlessness, that utter smallness, is what draws so many to the ocean, and what may just as powerfully repel others. The search for the good does not have an end. At some level within each of us we bear a question, always being asked and ever being answered. At times we have a sense of comfortable certitude and then without warning, we are tossed into a tailspin, with no idea which way is up.

Perhaps, the keystone idea in the previous paragraphs is about what is "good." We may all want a good life for each of our children, but what "good" means in depth and detail is more than a little debatable. A life dedicated to the acquisition of wealth and things or to hedonistic pleasure might be called "good," but such a life likely would look *wildly* different from a life given over to the joy of service to others or to contemplation and study. Even greater confusion results when we depart from the big life questions to consider questions that are more modest and practical. What is a "good" major in college? What groups are "good" to join? What is "good" to do in caring for a spouse, a child or an aging parent? We might also consider what is "good" to do in more immediate circumstances as well, like in the classical hypothetical situation where one is asked to choose between saving one's own life and saving the lives of five strangers from a speeding train. Considerations of any of these questions regarding the "good" do not exist in isolation. If we consider whether it is defensible for a police officer to use lethal force in a questionable circumstance, details of that circumstance can be considered in light of larger demands on the police officer, the human being killed, and the wider communities touched by the event.

The ultimate end or aim of an action is a worthy object of contemplation since such a thing can help us place in larger context any action or idea that we might assess from an ethical perspective. Ethicists refer to the ultimate ends sought by action or by a set of actions as the *telos*. It can also be useful to think about times when the ends sought by an action categorically *do not* matter. Sometimes "good" intentions are not sufficient for something to be "good," especially in terms of a given outcome.

What we need, it would seem, is some idea for making "good" decisions big and small; some idea or standard that can function as firmament or foundation for such decision-making. The larger problem, really the *huge* problem for us in this task, is choice. Ends matter, or perhaps they do not, but in the final analysis what really interests us in ethics, in leadership and in heroism is the making of a choice: a choice to save (or not), a choice to lead (or not), a choice to invest in another or one's self (or not). As we shall soon see, Aristotle understood this only too well and yet for all his wisdom, not to mention the wisdom of the many other sages, it might seem we are still often uncertain of anything related to what is good.

In *Man's Search for Meaning*, Viktor Frankl (2006) recounts his experiences as a prisoner in a Nazi concentration camp. More to the point, he tells us about his survival strategy having emerged from the ordeal, scarred, but wiser and more at peace within himself. As the title of his work indicates, meaning was what helped him navigate through a place that precipitated death daily. He could not cling to the idea of seeing his wife again, as the greater likelihood was that she would be gone, lost to the ovens of a concentration camp. He reasoned instead that he had a body of psychiatric scholarship he needed to attend to, that he had things to say that only he could say. He *had* to survive because he had a book to write, and that book was becoming more crucial daily as he learned about himself and his fellow humans in the midst of unspeakable horror. What he learned was that meaning was a life raft, but that meaning's power is indelibly tied to choice. He tells about a fellow inmate's connection to meaning through choice. Word had come to inmates that the Allies were making progress and might liberate the camp in the next few months. The inmate dreamt that they would come on a certain day and pinned all his hope on his dream's precision. Frankl counseled him not to fixate on the dream's predicted date for liberation, but to hold fast to the idea of the freedom to come. When the Allies got bogged down by German resistance, the inmate's hope faded. The predicted day of liberation came and went, and in the smallest hours of the next day, the inmate's ordeal ended. He died in his sleep, seemingly of a broken spirit. There is also the conversation Anthony de Mello (Braswell, 2018: 67) writes about where two old friends who had been in a Nazi concentration camp together were reunited. One friend asks the other if he had forgiven the Nazis, to which his friend replied that he had. The friend who had asked the question maintained that he had not, that he still hated them, to which his friend gently replied, "In that case, they still have you in prison."

We live, eat, sleep and die for meaning, but meaning, its cultivation and its use is a choice. It is not sufficient to consider what choices are good. We need to be clear as to larger ideas regarding the good, and then choose to live by (or not) these larger ideas. Although there are a considerable number of normative ethical frameworks, we can think of most of them as falling into four broad categories: virtue ethics, utilitarianism or consequentialism, deontology or non-consequentialism, and what we might call an ethic of care.

We begin our discussion with virtue ethics, specifically with a look at the Nicomachean Ethics of Aristotle. We begin there because, as we shall see, the other major schools of thought can be seen as having some measure of roots in Aristotle's arguments. In this discussion, keep an eye peeled for the use of different grounding ideas, ideas that give us the sense of something solid against which to push ourselves into the tossing current of life and all its choices.

Virtue Ethics

Although it is true that to some extent, the current state of philosophy has increasingly become a blend of both Eastern and Western philosophical traditions, we still tend to think of Greece as our philosophical stellar nursery or North Star. Like the astronomical phenomenon, certain places and times seem particularly fertile, able to produce a far greater share of philosophical stars than might otherwise be their lot. Such a place was the city-states of ancient Greece, particularly Athens, beginning around 2,600 years ago and lasting for nearly 300 years. Philosophers like Pythagoras, Socrates, Plato and Aristotle were the stars of their day. It is from two of the most lauded philosophers among them, Plato and Aristotle, that we receive the idea of virtue ethics. Many of the essential parts of the virtue ethical argument were present in the work of earlier thinkers; a similar view was presented by Confucius in China, for example. For this treatment we will focus primarily on Aristotle's formulation. Specifically, we will turn to the Nicomachean Ethics of Aristotle (e.g., 2019), a work containing Aristotle's formulation of virtue.

Aristotle's point of departure for his Ethics, in fact the very first words of the book, assert that every art and every practice strive for some kind of "good." A good carpenter makes good tables; a good table fulfills its function well. A master's bridle is to be preferred to a bridle made by a novice. But hold on just a moment: one might immediately protest that some confusion had arisen from vagueness in defining the term "good." Saying a thing like a table or a bridle is good tells us nothing about how we should live our lives.

If things can be "good," and if people can also be good, then there must be an innate nature in those things and those people that is objectively identifiable as "good-ness." We make choices for the sake of something, typically avoiding pain and seeking pleasure, and it is this something that interests Aristotle. The fact that we choose things or people (and not other things or people) points directly to the existence of some inherent goodness in those things or people. In some cases, the good nature of a thing or person is innate. In other instances, it can be cultivated. Recognizing the nature of the good in any given context is, for Aristotle, noble. Cultivating that good for a community is the highest nobility. This, of course, begs the question of what he means by "good," especially if it varies across contexts. "Good" is anything that advances eudaimonia (ευδαιμονια) or human flourishing. Eudaimonia is both an inward state of virtue and any activity that cultivates the flourishing of human life. We are conditioned by nature to have a propensity for good, in no small measure in terms of how we experience pleasure and pain.

It seems we crave a firmament or foundation beneath our feet; almost without thinking about it we desire some kind of an objective standard. Aristotle finds his grounding in the body of the hypothetical person in possession of practical reason (φρονησις, phronesis). This is the same person often relied upon in Western jurisprudence (e.g., in tort law, United States v. Carroll Towing Co.; search and seizure, Terry v. Ohio; see also Phair, 2017; see Gardner, 2015 for an erudite treatment regarding British law; see Fernandez, 2017 regarding defamation and the reasonable person standard in Australia). Such a firmament is both confusing and enlightening in some instances (see Vitiello, 2010). In Liebeck v. McDonald's Restaurants (1994), the infamous "hot coffee" case, for example, the reasonable person referenced by the jury in their decision seems to defy reason itself, handing Ms. Liebeck a small fortune because her coffee was "too hot" and yet, when the facts of the case are arranged in a certain way, the reasonable person standard seems to work precisely as Aristotle intended. In actuality, her precipitating actions were reasonable and her suffering – being scalded to the point of requiring long-term painful care – was considerable. Some argue that as a standard, it may be the best we can manage, at least for legal purposes (Vitiello, 2010). Then again, a reasonable person standard in a vastly diverse human community is fraught with shortcomings (see, e.g., Friedland, 2016).

The good, then, is that which is done by good people. Well, how do we know *who* is good, then?! They do good things, of course. This, you can tell, is circular reasoning and does not help us determine how to live. In actuality, Aristotle's argument is not circular, but it does require a little clarification. The person with phronesis (practical reason) acts with understanding as well as a set of virtuous traits. The starting point, then, of virtue, is having phronesis which includes the idea that knowledge is the beginning and choice is pivotal. The virtuous person must (1) act from *knowledge*; (2) must *choose* to do right; and (3) that action must be the result of a constant and unchanging *nature* within the person. A good state is one led by good politicians who work to further eudaimonia by cultivating potential of virtue within each citizen. Virtues are practiced. As youths, our good habits and actions lead to a more virtuous character, much like practicing a guitar makes one a better guitar player.

What, then, can we learn from the cultivated state of character? What knowledge might we seek to pursue in order to choose nobly and thus possess virtue? For Aristotle the answer lies in the middle. Virtue is parabolic: cowardice (acting cowardly in response to fear) is not virtuous. Hubris or rashness (being overconfident in a dangerous situation) is likewise not virtuous. Courage, however, now *that* is something. Doing a daring thing like a dangerous action in wartime despite being afraid is virtuous according to Aristotle. Often, we find virtue to be a point between two extreme attributes. Courage as an example highlights the importance of knowledge (one knows there is danger) and choice (one acts despite it). Even something like truthfulness can be found at the midpoint between boastfulness and false modesty.

Aristotle recognizes, though, that context also matters. The midpoint between two vices is not necessarily always the most virtuous action. Sometimes it is perfectly reasonable to be more afraid than at other times. One of the authors, for example, is not a fan of spiders. Collecting and freeing a spider from one's bathroom is not a task that is equal in virtue for the authors. For one of us to free a spider it takes rather more courage than the other. Laziness and excessive exercise are two opposite poles and are thus vices, making the proper amount of exercise the virtuous or golden mean. What is a proper amount of exercise for one person is not necessarily indicative of what is proper for someone else. Someone just beginning an exercise routine after extensive surgery should proceed gently but not lazily. To be sure, our patient should not leap out of bed and into the CrossFit gym seeking to set any world records, but neither should he undertake his recovery in lax fashion. Finally, Aristotle recognizes that the extremes regarding vices are not necessarily equal. Sometimes one extreme is closer to the virtue than another. It is difficult and at times can seem impossible to find a virtuous balance or golden mean in many situations, which is why seeking the cultivated state of character he talked about is important. Aristotle is clear that finding and holding such a balance is in no way easy. He compares it to holding a boat in place against the treacherous tide, which might sound familiar. Again, it is a thing to be practiced lifelong, a thing to be cultivated by preceding generations and conveyed to following generations, usually through the action of parents and the state.

Utilitarianism, Teleology or Consequentialism

Aristotle employed the idea of pleasure and pain as evidence of our naturalized sense of the good. This natural capacity for good is a keystone idea for his argument about eudaimonia, and thus his larger arguments about virtue which we just reviewed. Instead of pleasure and pain serving in something of a predictive role, Utilitarians like Jeremy Bentham firmly fixed pleasure and pain at the very epicenter of their reasoning. Pleasure *is* ethical, and pain *is* unethical, simply put. More specifically, the grounding used by utilitarians for understanding right action is the idea of maximizing pleasure and minimizing pain for the most people, and the likelihood of that pleasure or pain occurring following the action in question. Pleasure/pain consequences are what makes a thing ethical or not, which is why it is called "consequentialism." For any given action, then, we would think about the value of the pleasure or pain that would likely follow the act, and the likelihood of that pleasure or pain arising. We would also think about the same things – the value and likelihood – for each person impacted by the act (DeValve, Garland, & Wright, 2018).

For example, if we are contemplating whether it is right for a person to leap into an icy pond to save a child, the potential hero's action involves both pain (swimming in icy water) and potential pleasure should the hero succeed and receive the gratitude of the child, his parents and perhaps a wider community. To this we would add the pain experienced by the child, which could be extreme as it might include death, the pain experienced by the parents as well as the pleasure of their child being rescued. There is also the pain associated with the possible death of the hero and the pain experienced by the community at large as well as the pleasure of having both child and hero alive to contribute to the community.

One of the more flawed aspects of Bentham's formulation of utilitarianism is that it is, in his view, perfect. In the end, though, utilitarianism fails for a larger and more basic reason: we are just not that simple a species. More factors than pain and pleasure work upon and within us, and merely redefining all of our nuance and immanence as pleasure and pain denies our complexity and potential for monstrous deeds and acts of staggering beauty and kindness.

Deontology or Non-Consequentialism

It speaks to our complexity as a species that we might identify some things in the scope of our human experience that seem, well, just plain right or just plain wrong in and of themselves. Some of Immanuel Kant's acolytes, citing his "Formula of Humanity," might argue, for example, that killing another human being is absolutely indefensible regardless of circumstances (although Kant himself would not argue that all killing is indefensible – he was an advocate of the death penalty and of killing in self-defense [see, e.g., Kleingeld, 2019]), not in wartime, not in self-defense, certainly not for even the most extraordinary profit. No outcome can justify killing in the eyes of such Kantians. In the archetypal ethical example, we have a time machine, a pistol and detailed information where the child Adolf Hitler will be on a certain day in history. No other options aside from his murder are possible. Would it be defensible to shoot a young Hitler in order to prevent the bloody conflagration that became World War II? Add to your contemplations that a conservative estimate of the lives lost during World War II in Europe is approximately 25 million. To this we might add a few other consequences from that single life. First, national socialist reasoning enjoyed amplification through him and led in turn to the suffering and death of many human beings, for example in Spain. The fallout of the European collision led to the Cold War and, thus, to the spin-off conflicts like the Korean "police action," the Vietnam conflict and the Soviet invasion of Afghanistan. We might continue and throw in more recent costs, including the American conflict in Afghanistan and Iraq; most likely there would not have been a Taliban if there hadn't been a Mujahidin. All told, we might reckon the cost of Adolf Hitler's life and leadership as being something to the tune of 40–50 million lives. Still, some would argue, the cost of executing one innocent child, even if that innocent child is the young Adolf Hitler, is simply too high. The consequences of killing young Adolf do not make the act of killing him acceptable, and in fact their contemplation itself is nonsensical.

We cannot know the consequences of changing an event in time. For these reasons we call this perspective non-consequentialism.

There are a set of things, then, that are universal, absolute duties or, as Kant put it, "categorical imperatives." We should act in ways that are compatible with creating a kind of universal law. If you toss your burger wrapper out of your car window, it must be defensible in your view that everyone could do the same thing. Kant calls this the principle of moral universalism, often referred to as the Formula of Universal Law. If you feel you have a right to air, water, food or healthcare, then it must be the case that everyone is so entitled.

Viewing the provision of air, water, food and healthcare as rights rooted in Kant's Formula of Humanity also speaks to the idea of the existence of fundamental and unqualified duties, duties that have nothing to do with pleasure or with eudaimonia. We might take from these examples the idea that human situations compel other humans to action, that meaningfully addressing human need is a categorical imperative. This categorical requirement to address human need stems from Kant's assertion that human beings are ends in themselves and can never be viewed as a means to an end, no matter what that end may be. "Using" a person to achieve, well, anything, violates Kant's Formula of Humanity. The person used *is* the end and what is more, he or she is an end that supersedes all other possible ends. In other words, the ends never justify the means if the means are people. One of us included a problem in our ethics class. At issue was the question: since human beings aren't perfect, no system we create can be absolutely perfect. Given that reality, if we could successfully execute 10,000 Ted Bundys and other serial murders, resulting in many innocent victims being saved, at the expense of one innocent person being convicted and executed, would it be worth the cost? Asking for a show of hands, typically 95 percent of the class agreed that it would, indeed, be worth the cost. Asking the students in agreement to keep their hands held high, I then asked them if that one innocent person was their brother, sister, father, mother or even themselves, would they still support the required execution. As you might imagine, hands came down quickly, which illustrates Kant's point: you cannot be willing for someone else to suffer something you aren't willing to suffer (Braswell, McCarthy, & McCarthy, 2020).

The grounding of a deontological perspective is the idea of the categorical imperative that stems from humans as ends. If you recall, Aristotle made the point relatively early on in the *Ethics*, that some things are not "meanable" in the sense of a golden mean's virtue balance. Some things are just not okay. Aristotle seems to indicate that the wrongness is evident in the words themselves, that no room exists for adultery or murder. One cannot philander correctly or murder tastefully. This inherent wrongness in these things or the inherent goodness of adhering to categorical duties is the firmament on which Kant plants his feet.

Ethics of Care

It is a sound critique of much of Western philosophy that it is composed of the voices of white men. It goes without saying, of course, that the dominance of men in philosophy was in no way a function of their corner on the market of capacity. Women and People of Color lived on the margins of academia until relatively recently and to our collective detriment. With the amplification of feminine voices and Voices of Color came a new fertility and relevance. It is in this new creative fertility that an ethic of care, compassion and love finds its most potent roots. There are a number of voices that contribute to the idea of an ethic of care, including Nell Noddings, but we will look at just two, and only briefly: Carol Gilligan and Simone Weil.

The Aristotelian idea of eudaimonia is not altogether alien to an ethic of care. Often the Greek is mistranslated to refer to happiness and, although the particulars vary, both Aristotle and care ethicists intend something more radiant and expansive than simple happiness. The ethics of care also share something with deontological arguments: the idea that people are ends in themselves. Care ethics, though, tend to focus on and develop this idea more fully than Kant or Kantian ethicists do. The attention to needs that come from the idea of people as ends in themselves operates as an objective standard for acting or critiquing actions in a general sense. An ethic of love, though, takes an individualized angle on the idea of need and human value. Deontological arguments and love–ethical arguments share a recognition of the fundamental value of human life and the motive and force that come from human need, but that is where their similarities end. They view humanity in strikingly different ways. They attend to different levels of detail in the human experience, and as a result they make different assertions about what human need invites or compels.

Recall our mention of the principle of moral universalism. It is a generalizable principle that does little more than assert the existence of a generalized universal duty. Everyone is equally situated in Kant's framework; rather, we might say that social location is irrelevant. A duty is a duty is a duty, and that duty is universal to everyone. Everyone has the same duties, but also everyone has the same rights. This is egalitarian and, to many, attractive. An ethic of care, however, zooms in and examines where people find themselves in terms of their networks, and speaks in terms of particulars. It centers not only on attending to need or responding to suffering, but also actualizing the other, the object of ethical action.

Carol Gilligan (e.g., 1993) offers us what she calls the "care perspective." Although she is careful not to correlate this perspective with womanhood as such, it is the result of the contemplation of the feminine voice in questions of human psychological ontology, phenomenology and development that had historically excluded feminine ideas. When she entered the academy, Piaget, Freud, Erikson and Kohlberg – all men – represented the major theoretical influences on developmental psychology. These thinkers bore within their theories something of an assumption of the ideal individual as autonomous and independent, able to succeed according to objective measures of cognitive and ethical performance. In rather sharp contrast, Gilligan's theorizing is rooted in the idea that humans are relational and responsive beings. Women tend to, but all of us could, see ourselves and our world in terms of our relationships to others, and that need or suffering compels response from others in that common human experience of having been the object of caring action at some point in life (Gilligan, 1993). We are possible as beings only because of the care of others, and it is this caring, rooted in our interdependence, that provides the grounding of her ethical framework. It isn't a categorical imperative that she identifies in the act of caring because it is in "choosing" to care that gives it life and force.

Simone Weil is not typically viewed as an ethical theorist, although her ideas are richly relevant to an ethic of care/love. Like Gilligan, Weil's grounding is tied to human interdependence and connection and, like Gilligan, she recognized the power of the choice to care, the will-to-love if you prefer, to be at the heart of political responsibility. Although she came from a privileged home full of learning and scholarly pursuits, she sought the chance to work in factories in order to understand the plight of the underclass. What she saw there changed her in a profound way. Never a particularly healthy person herself, the physical tests of the factory wore on her but not more than the emotional and psychological burdens of menial and monotonous work. She did not remain long in the factory. Later she found joy in hard labor on a farm near Marseilles and then committed herself utterly to the reestablishment of the French Republic after the Nazi occupation.

Simone Weil left us a wealth of wisdom in her writings, but for our current purposes in terms of understanding an ethical framework founded on love and caring, she offers us a particular insight that deserves some scrutiny, one that differs from both Kant's and Gilligan's grounding.

"There is in each human being," she writes, "something sacred. But it is not his...personality. It is him, this man, wholly and simply" (Weil, 2015a: 104). She points to a certain divinity within each human and argues that this divinity has a certain expectation that evil will not be done to it. When evil is done, a cry arises: "Why has this been done to me?" The cry invites others to action but does not necessarily compel it. Public education, she says, should facilitate both the means of expressing this cry and the authentic response to it that begins with silence and leads to compassionate action. The divine in us to which she points is very difficult to speak to in any objective way, even though she calls for a society organized around it.

Simone Weil gives us another idea related to what we have discussed but of measurably greater value for our discussion to come. In a number of her writings she speaks of "reading." Reading is an act whereby someone perceives aspects of the world around her: the sea, the sky, the pen skipping on the page (Weil, 2015b: 23), but that perception does not occur in isolation. The perception of particular parts of the universe is in us, rich with meaning. Words on a page, just squiggles of ink on wood pulp really, have the capacity to punch as forcefully as a champion boxer, perhaps an example of the pen often being mightier than the sword. The universe around us operates on and within us, triggering action almost without our permission or participation, like yanking a scorched hand back from a hot fire. The thing is, she tells us, that we are not without the capacity to change appearances, how we read the world, and, thus, to change how we act in response to our understanding of the world. We can transform the meaning we perceive. She wrote much of the body of her works just before and during World War II and in fact, she did not live to see its conclusion. She speaks of the reading of rifle fire and explosions, only too well aware of their consequences. Yet she asserts that we have a measure of control over meaning. Someone reads a circumstance: danger is perceived. The meaning of the circumstance, the danger, though, is ours to make or remake, and it is in this choice to remake meaning, to read wisely, that heroes arise.

Normative Ethics: Conclusion

These ethical arguments and discussions are useful to a degree, sometimes, and some more often than others. Some operate like guardrails and like footholds; they are pinned to something that seems to give us a sense of reference; some aid in our climb toward good. Other ethical explorations seek to shape our attention and deepen our awareness of our own beauty and vulnerability. Practical reason that cultivates eudaimonia, the net balance or golden mean of pleasure and pain, the idea of humans as ends in themselves, or that human need compels actualizing action, each is held up by their advocates as being the most important in determining the good in an action. We seem to crave that rooted rock against which to push as we move into the unpredictable surf of our life experiences. Perhaps, instead of firmament on which to push into the surf, we should seek to help each other become better swimmers.

Virtue ethics, utilitarianism and deontological ethics are useful for analyzing some kinds of action, but there is something in the idea of heroism almost by definition that transcends and leaves behind any ethical analysis. In some ways heroism as an idea diminishes ethical claims about the universal good, precisely because it calls us to act in ways beyond what any ethical standard might assert is expectable of us. Heroic action is often supra-ethical, which is precisely what makes it heroism. If it were deducible from a calculus or dictated by a categorical imperative, it would cease to be extraordinary. It is almost as if the use of a universal, objective standard, almost by its nature, banishes heroism to the margins of human activity, rendering it an exception to the rule. An ethic of care, however, not only reclaims and celebrates heroism; it makes it attainable to everyone who is willing to swim against the tide of routine and tradition.

Leadership Theories

In something of a contrast to normative ethical theories, theories about leadership tend to be somewhat more ontological, meaning that they seek to explain a thing in the human experience. These theories grow out of the nearly ubiquitous, but often exceptional, circumstance where one human steps forward from among others and acts in some fashion that resolves some pressing, perhaps even ultimate, concern that faces them. The leader need not be a formally designated one, though she or he may be; such leaders may not be physically or intellectually mighty, but they may be. One traditional definition of power (Dahl, 1957) is the ability of Person A to get Person B to do what Person A wants done. Iconic American army general and former president Dwight Eisenhower is purported to have modified this definition somewhat: "leadership is the art of getting someone else to do something you want done because he wants to do it." It was between the spasms of suffering we call the Great Depression and World War II when Chester Barnard wrote his iconic tome (Barnard, 1938/1971). Barnard reminds us all that organizations exist in at least two dimensions: formal and informal. A leader need not be a chief, CEO, president or even from a middling rank within the formal structure. Indeed, a leader may not even realize she or he is a leader at all. Burns (1978) tells us, in fact, that leadership is often observed but poorly understood. Although his observation is now more than 40 years old, it remains as true now as then. Almost everyone can think of a situation where they have experienced something they understand to be "leadership," a moment where someone took charge, rose up or stood out and, through words or deeds, led a group to the accomplishment of some goal.

Viewing leadership in these terms, it seems all too easy to regard leadership and heroism as nearly synonymous. After all, both leaders and heroes do stand out from a group and may go to extraordinary circumstances to achieve their aims. Although leaders can be heroes and vice versa, we understand it to be a potentially grave mistake to assume leaders are by definition heroes and vice versa. The space between the two is rather more evident when we examine the phenomena themselves: leader*ship* and hero*ism*. Even from what we have already examined regarding heroism, the gap between the two phenomena is evident. Achilles, for example, was without doubt a leader, but his example is somewhat harder to cast today as heroism. Don Quixote is a tragic hero in both literary terms and in terms of his ideological example, but it would be a stretch to say he exhibited capable leadership to any great degree. Let us look a little more closely at thought related to leadership as a phenomenon.

As we have already indicated, leadership theories seek to describe the phenomenon others, often non-leaders, perceive when a particular individual takes charge, embraces a challenge and leads. It is something of an awkward assumption, though, to assume that just because people have led that there is a discernible and discrete thing such as leader*ship*. The search for extraterrestrial life, for example, for the most part has operated from the perspective of the one known instance of sentient life arising in the universe: our own. Exo-biologists and planetary scientists must resist the only-too-natural tendency to theorize about life elsewhere in terrestrial terms. In our search in the solar system and elsewhere for sentience, "earth*ship*" (e.g., the idea of the "Goldilocks zone") is a reasonable trait for which to look. But earthship as a framework for looking for extraterrestrial intelligence necessarily channels our search away from places where other iterations of sentience may exist.

Our aim here will be to review briefly some of the main theories regarding leadership as a human phenomenon. These theories have arisen over a far shorter time scale than has normative ethical theories. It would seem reasonable, then, to think about leadership as a single dialogue, dividable into theoretical parts – trait theory, behavioral theory, contingency theory – and what we might call postmodern humanist theory. Within this arc of thought we will present what many call leadership styles (e.g., democratic, laisse-faire, autocratic, transformational, primal and servant), many of which represent polar opposite approaches to the challenge of leading.

It serves us well, we think, to begin with an important observation about how for the most part, contemporary leadership theories arose. Contemporary formal thinking about leadership is part of a larger organizational and administrative theoretical project; thinkers from Woodrow Wilson to Robert Denhardt contemplated the nature of how human organizations should operate. Some, like Chester Barnard, Fredrick Winslow Taylor and Peter Drucker, came from a for-profit perspective and contemplated business organizations. Others like Wilson, Denhardt and Paul Appleby concerned themselves chiefly with public organizations and their operation. Contemporary leadership theories almost exclusively operate from the perspective of the maximization of organizational effectiveness. A good bit of leadership theorizing might be fruitfully understood as the flipside of thought about motivation in organizations. As such, that bit of thought can be dehumanizing and inclined to detract from our pursuit for insight into the morphology of the ordinary hero.

One last point is necessary here. As a result of the how and why of contemporary leadership theories, there tended to be, at least into the later part of the twentieth century, a blurring of the distinction between leadership and management. We will talk about a "managerial grid" and "participatory management," for example, in our discussion on leadership. We do not operate from the assumption, though, that leadership and management are often close to the same thing organizationally. One classic formulation posits that management refers to "doing things right," whereas leadership means "doing the right thing." This distinction might be described in terms of function versus vision. A manager, say, a police sergeant, knows how to properly make an arrest and may well be adroit at teaching the finer points of the process, whereas a leader knows when arrest as a tool is fruitful in a given situation.

Trait Theory

The earliest and probably most primitive approach to leadership does not deal directly with leadership styles much at all. Leadership itself, the capacity to leap to the front of the pack and bring people together to confront a challenge, might be a trait; it might be an indelible characteristic. One is born with it, some say. We might be better served to identify some more particular attributes if such is the case. We might also take some examples for inspiration: Ronald Reagan was tall, handsome, charismatic and among some groups he is still deeply admired as a president. His nickname, "the great communicator," is fodder for our contemplations. He was effective not merely at relaying information but at keeping an audience rapt and even drawing them into a way of thinking that was not necessarily originally their own.

We might also think of someone like Winston Churchill. He was not tall and it would stretch credulity to call him handsome. He disliked Mohandas Gandhi immensely and, although this may not be evidence of racism as such, it is at least evidence of the depth of his imperialist feelings. At the moment when Britain truly needed him, when the Nazi German military behemoth stared hungrily at them across the narrow English Channel and the Luftwaffe unleashed strategic bombing on the civilian population, he was the stalwart and resolute presence on the radio and in the chambers of Parliament that the British people needed.

Traits like courage, presence, intelligence, capacity for autonomous action, even attractiveness all have been correlated with the idea of leadership. Traits, at least some traits, are either possessed by a person or they are not. There is no surgery that can implant courage or charisma. Also, we must recognize that for a trait to be of leadership relevance, it needs to be expressed behaviorally. And as we will discover, what traits matter may well vary according to the context of a given situation.

Behavioral Theories of Leadership

As traits like courage or insight or panache must be realized in actual outward behavior in order to be relevant for leadership in an organization, thinking about leadership naturally turns to an examination of leadership behavior. This turn was influenced by two additional currents of the time. First, the work of B.F. Skinner turned psychological pursuits toward a cognitive contemplation of action, emphasizing behavior over concerns regarding internal motivation. Second, it seemed to many that the world stage had been set for a collision of ideologies: democracy, fascism and communism. Each side had to make its strongest case to the rest of humanity in order to prevail. As the 1930s wound down, a contest to resolve the collision seemed inevitable.

Inevitable or not, such a collision is precisely what happened. In steps Kurt Lewin. He and his colleagues (Lewin, Lippitt, & White, 1939) examined experimentally the impact of different leadership styles on the aggressive and apathetic behavior of young boys. Three leadership styles were employed in their design: democratic leadership, laissez-faire leadership and authoritarian leadership. Although the results were by no means straightforward, Lewin and his colleagues concluded that democratic leadership produced less aggression and less apathy and was thus innately more desirable an approach to leading humans in organizations. Lewin and a good portion of his Western audience surmised that participatory leadership in most organizational contexts made very good sense. Involving workers in the process of making work-related decisions seemed to increase their sense of wellbeing and, perhaps, even their productivity. Findings by Kahn and Katz (1968) seemed to indicate that even across multiple contexts, participatory involvement of workers seemed to yield greater productivity in comparison to leaders who tended to have a more task-oriented approach to leadership.

It turns out, though, that productivity under participatory management did not always prove to be better in all circumstances. Context matters it seems, more than Lewin might have assumed. What was known as "The Michigan Studies" was an examination of different leadership styles and their impact on effectiveness and worker satisfaction. Led by Rensis Likert, the guiding assumption was that democratic leadership would prove to be both more effective and more positively received. World War II had silenced only one of the three ideological systems whose collision of claims gave shape to the musings and misery of the twentieth century. The Cold War would prove to be an intense contest between the two remaining ideologies, and not a few social scientists were keen to leap into formation. Likert's examination of leader styles in a variety of organizations (e.g., Likert, 1967) revealed that, indeed, participatory management was superior not only in terms of employee satisfaction and motivation but also in relation to work product quality. The catch was that aside from the collaborative, supportive and participatory leader, other organizational conditions needed also to be present such as collaborative communication throughout the organization, leader competence and upwardly adjusted performance benchmarks along with participatory leadership in order for this approach to yield its potential benefits. One big corollary of the Michigan Studies was that leader behavior, important though it may be, was not in itself sufficient to bring about the motivational and performance-related outcomes desired. In fact, findings also indicated that leaders fell into two general categories: those concerned for workers and those more concerned for the product or process. Another oversized research project, this one the Ohio State Studies, likewise found similar results to regarding leader behavior. Instead of Likert's terms, they used the terms "initiating structure" to refer to concern for production and "consideration" to indicate concern for people.

Following the Michigan and Ohio State studies, Blake and Mouton (1966) developed a conceptual model of management that they called the "managerial grid." Along one axis is "concern for people" and along the other is "concern for production." The grid produces five managerial types: at the lower right corner of the grid is the high-production-low-people "produce or perish" manager; across from it at the upper left corner is the low-production-high-people "country club" manager. In the lower left corner where both people concern and production concern are low is the "impoverished" manager. In the upper right corner, with high concern for both people and production is the "team manager." Finally, in the middle of the grid balanced between the two axes is the "middle of the road" manager. As one might infer from the names given, the team manager was thought to be preferable in most circumstances, although Blake and Mouton were careful to observe that context really does matter in determining which managerial style works best.

Another project took this idea of the people/production grid one step further and deepened the conversation about context. Hersey and Blanchard (1969) took Blake and Mouton's grid almost as it was, but instead of viewing it in terms of semi-static styles, they argued that it represented something of a pathway for some for-profit entrepreneurial managers. In the beginning, an entrepreneurial organization would be production-focused, and so the leader needed to live more in the lower right corner in what Hersey and Blanchard call "telling" activities. As the organization becomes more established, concern for employees' growth and development necessitates a move toward the upper right of the grid, toward what Hersey and Blanchard (1969) call the "selling" end of the grid. Once the organization is well established and a crop of managers are cultivated (though they may not have the vision needed to lead), the entrepreneur can move toward the upper left, or "participating" corner. Finally, once both product and people are fully ready, the entrepreneur can move toward the lower left, or "delegating" approach. The maturity of the organization itself plays an important role in the contemplation of context.

Yet another study raised important questions about a nearly sacrosanct psychological theory: Abraham Maslow's (1943) hierarchy of needs. Most everyone is familiar with Maslow's hierarchy; needs related to immediate safety are more immediately pressing than needs for food and water, which are in turn more important than the human need for esteem, and onward to the pinnacle of the model, self-actualization. Geert Hofstede (1991), however, found that the hierarchy as Maslow proposed it appeared to be culturally specific and that aside from safety and biological needs, non-European communities often had ultimate concerns that were significantly different from what Maslow's model portrayed. Related to this kind of contextual variable is another theoretical development that followed from the Ohio State studies. Scholarship by Robert House and Terrence Mitchell (House & Mitchell, 1975) indicates that the effective leadership style in any given organizational situation is a function of what is needed to cultivate employee empowerment. House and Mitchell called their leadership model "path-goal" leadership. Effective leaders should set the goals for the team and, knowing how to empower the particular employees they had, they would clarify the path to achieve that goal. In essence, path-goal leadership is understandable as something of a slightly humanized behaviorist approach to leading, varying according to employee preferences (see also DeValve, 2007). If context matters so much, then it deserves formal theoretical consideration regarding leadership. Thus, we have contingency theories of leadership.

Contingency Theories

For our purposes here it is sufficient to discuss the big theory among contingency theories: that offered by Fred Fiedler. A native Austrian, he immigrated to the United States before World War II and served in the army. After the war he returned to the Chicago area where he had been living and completed his education in clinical psychology. His experiences in the army and working with the Veterans' Administration led him to take on the task of studying leadership in the navy.

Fiedler's thinking about leadership very much took what had been going on in leadership theorizing more generally as a point of departure. Specifically, the task-versus-relationship dynamic present in the Michigan and Ohio State studies was fore in his thinking. At the same time, he well recognized what we have already discussed – that organizational and personal variables also went into the success of a leader's attempt to lead. His theory (e.g., Fiedler, 2006), then, really needed to have two semi-distinct limbs.

First, he set out to create an instrument that could be used psychometrically to determine the task/relationship preference for any given leader or potential leader. His measure for task/relationship preference was based on the idea of a least-preferred co-worker: how willing one was to work with one's least-preferred co-worker was a sensible measure for how relationship-oriented one might be. Thus, he had the first limb.

Second, he needed to create something of a conceptual model that would help determine how and when someone was relatively effective at wielding power in a social setting. Whether that setting be an advanced engineering shop like the "Skunk Works" or a tightly controlled combat situation, leadership as he conceived it was about the ability of a leader to get others to do something. Think, for example of what has come to be called the *"Birkenhead Drill"* (named after the HMS *Birkenhead* in honor of the soldiers on her), or the actions of what the Soviets called the "liquidators," cleaning up the deadly debris of the Chernobyl disaster. Well, Fiedler theorized that the significant organizational and personal variables could be summed up with three axes: leader–member relations, task structure and position power. Regarding leader–member relations, a given leader might enjoy the personal confidence of her subordinates, or she may not; leader–member relations can be good or not so good. Depending on its inherent nature, a task might be highly structured, or such structure may not be fully possible. Assembling a Big Mac is a straightforward task; writing a novel or designing a plane is not such a straightforward task. Finally, the formal power and status that attend a given position can vary, and widely. An army general wields considerable power over her soldiers, whereas an academic dean holds relatively less formal authority. Good/poor leader–member relations, high/low task structure and high/low formal authority, each aligned along one axis in three dimensions, end up creating a cube with eight subsections. Fiedler referred to these eight sections as octants.

Taking the two limbs together, then, we can conceive of a whole smattering of leaders and then theorize about their relative effectiveness. A task-focused leader with high formal position power but poor leader–member relations leading a group tasked with completing a highly complicated task is unlikely to fare well; the same is likely for a relationship-focused leader with very good leader–member relations who is tasked with performing the very structured – and crucial – task of assaulting a beach. A task-focused, empowered leader tasked with leading a group to complete a straightforward task is likely to succeed, as is a leader who is relationship-focused and not as reliant upon formal authority or excessive prestige charged with leading a group of experts asked to achieve a highly sophisticated task over several years.

The Postmodern Humanist Turn

There is a dynamic in the development of contemporary leadership thought that mirrors an important element present in the wider body of administrative theorizing. This dynamic is more particularly present in thought related to for-profit organizations, although it is not without its presence in public administration as well (e.g., Osborne & Gaebler, 1992). This dynamic relates to the ordering of organizational priorities. It has been assumed that for businesses, profit was the most important measure of success. It all comes down to the bottom line, and of course cash is king. At first, owners *were* the only managers and workers were merely expensive, but replaceable, moving parts in the machine. Train lines and beer distribution saw the first professional managers who did not own the means of production (Wren, 2005). The stage was set for the labor struggles that pocked the nineteenth and early twentieth centuries. Frederick Winslow Taylor (2014) sought to make peace between labor and management, arguing they both sought the same thing at the end of the day: success in the form of profit. Still, his scientific management could hardly be seen as softening the conditions of the worker beyond a minimal level. It was not that long ago (Senge, 2006), in fact, that the argument that people were *as* important as profit or that people were the very thing that assured profit was convincingly made.

In much the same fashion, the ground was not prepared for anything akin to a people-equal argument, let alone a people-first argument before the end of the twentieth century, but come it did. Influenced by postmodernism more generally, itself shaped in part by the introduction of Eastern philosophical ideas, a number of thinkers began to assert that although profit is indeed important, the people within the organization should be the central concern for leaders. We will discuss three relatively recent theoretical arguments that can be seen as dethroning the idea of production or profit as king and place the person fully at the center of a leader's concern.

James McGregor Burns (1978) created, and others like Bass and Riggio (2006), and Tichy and Devanna (1997) developed, the idea of transformational leadership. *Transactional* leadership operates as something of a counterpoint for thinking about transformational leadership. The transactional leader would take something of a path-goal behaviorist approach to leading. Transactional leadership works along the lines of an exchange process. The leader provides certain materials, services, opportunities and incentives, and indicates what output is expected in return. In this exchange, the locus of control remains extrinsic at least to a degree. In contrast, the transformational leader seeks to involve employees in the concerns of the organization by exposing them to, and, to a degree, involving them in, the contemplation of what once had been thought to be uniquely executive concerns. The transformational leader offers employees a compelling vision and then invites their involvement and, thus, their buy-in into a vision, which in turn leads to a kind of intrinsic motivation. Involvement in the concerns that confront the organization is the invitation to employees to invest themselves in common organizational concerns. Leaders retain their role at the pinnacle of the organization, but by involving employees in the larger concerns inside and outside the organization, they transform both the organization and employees, bringing both into higher states of capacity. One might think of transformational leadership as taking to its fullest extent Frederick Winslow Taylor's observation regarding the relationship between management and labor being guided by the same concerns. In the end, according to its advocates, the transformational leader is capable of both creating a deeper and more meaningful change and institutionalizing change within an organizational process.

Intrinsic motivation is a powerful device for leaders, but ethically speaking it is still problematic. Taking the idea of people-first leadership further is a movement called "primal leadership." Goleman (2005) and Boyatzis and McKee (2005) make a convincing argument regarding the importance of the emotional intelligence of leaders in relation to organizational outcomes. Influenced by developments in cortical neurology and by the recent movement toward mindfulness which is derived from Eastern, specifically Buddhist philosophy, primal leadership seeks to focus attention on the importance of being attuned to the emotional needs and rhythms of employees. The emotional intelligence of leaders is essential, primal leadership advocates contend, to helping employees grow and achieve according to their capacity. Primal leaders speak at length, for example, about concern regarding their employees' emotional states. They regard these states as essential to success, including the capacity to connect emotionally with their employees and avoiding emotional collisions. Primal leaders seek to understand the way the human limbic system and, in particular, the amygdala operate. The amygdala sits deep within the human brain. It is related to the experiencing of certain emotions, in particular fear and to the perception of those same emotions in others. When the amygdala is running hot and an employee is experiencing fear whether that fear is personal or professional, only a small emotional uptick can create dramatic, fear-driven results. Being sensitive to fear, working to calm and contextualize fears, is essential to helping employees be healthy and to achieve organizational goals.

The third and final approach to leadership we will discuss in this section is often referred to as "servant leadership." Servant leadership (Greenleaf, 2003) moves the people-first needle even further and seeks to center employees in the process of their actualization not only as an employee but as a person more generally. People, not profit or product, becomes the focal concern of organizational action. In fact, the purpose of leaders is to serve their employees. Employees are cultivated into leaders in their own right instead of being motivated to improve themselves through external incentives or intrinsic rewards. The goal of servant leadership is to cultivate each employee according to her or his highest capacity and only then are organizational interests served. Indeed, the servant leader would argue that by centering the people within the organization, the organization's interests are naturally fulfilled, not because they are motivated to serve the organization, but because they themselves are more robust, capable and actualized beings.

Greenleaf often gestures to a novel, *The Journey to the East*, by Herman Hesse as inspiration. In particular, he finds the character Leo to be of great importance. The main character has just joined a secretive league of travelers, and a group set off on a journey. The journey is a collective pilgrimage undertaken by league members, but very quickly it becomes clear that each member of the group has something of his own that he seeks. Along on the journey is a servant, Leo. He feeds them, gives them inspiration and even sings to them. Along the way, Leo leaves the group and the group falters. Spoiler alert: Leo isn't a servant at all. Rather, we should say that he *is* a servant, but he is *also* the leader of the shadowy league. By virtue of his job as leader he understands that his first duty to those he leads is to serve. And in his service, he comes to understand and to cultivate the capacities of his followers, and they come to understand themselves. What is more, in the very last pages of the novel the protagonist realizes that he and President Leo, though separate beings, were part of one larger truth, that the boundary between the two was decidedly less important than he had realized before.

Ethics and Leadership

So, what does all of this get us? We began the chapter with the assertion that theory was an eminently practical endeavor. We should be in search of something graspable we can show for our trouble. We also said that we should be very careful about making assumptions regarding the overlap of ethics, leadership and our understanding of heroism, that even if ideas about ethics and leadership can shed some light on what heroism is, we should never assume that heroism, leadership and ethics are even close to the same thing.

A first place to start looking for things practical is where ethics and leadership ideas overlap; consonance among ideas might well be a reasonable proxy for robustness. Virtue ethics and the trait theory of leadership, for example, seem to be natural bedfellows. Although some leadership traits, like communication skills, can readily be cultivated, other traits like Aristotle's phronesis are acquired almost glacially over time if they are ever truly acquired at all. It might be safe to assume that one of Aristotle's star pupils, Alexander III of Macedon (aka Alexander the Great), served as an example for Aristotle regarding leadership. It makes sense given what we have discussed already that all things exist and operate with a purpose in Aristotle's view; in a sense, things are inclined to move toward their ultimate state like mountains inevitably worn, dulled and in time made low by mighty water. Alexander might well have been a prime example for Aristotle: Alexander was destined to rule much of the known world by virtue of his suite of capacities. We might be well served, then, turning attention to the shoreline of *capacities and potentialities* that heroes have.

But Aristotle understood only too well the importance of context. Aristotle would probably argue that Alexander's capacity to rule was not necessarily total. His leadership potential and actuality were as much about those he conquered as they were about his own capacities (e.g., Levin, 1997). Virtue ethics as Aristotle framed it, then, also has some consonance with contingency theories of leadership, like Fred Fiedler's theory. *Context*, then, might well be an important concept for understanding heroism. Actions we might take to be heroic in one setting may be thought to be rather less heroic in others, and we would do well to pay attention to what is at work in context to determine heroism from something less noble.

Further, Aristotle's phronesis and eudaimonia often have been employed in an overly narrow way, as "intellect" and as "happiness" respectively. Such interpretations are faulty; it is not at all inappropriate to understand eudaimonia as "flourishing" or even as "actualization," which means that Aristotle's view on ethics can be connected (within limits) to any leadership theory that seeks to actualize organizational members or the clients they serve. It would be a stretch to take Aristotle to mean that everyone should be cultivated equally, that each person in an organization, in order to flourish, makes a natural and equal claim on everyone else. Some people just aren't as important or as capable as others in Aristotle's mind. Still, even if we were to accept Aristotle's biases (for example, women and slaves were very much less capable, and thus less valuable, than free men), the idea of *human actualization and flourishing* should be something we should seek to understand more fully with regard to heroism. Specifically, in the stories that follow, we should look very carefully into how the actions of heroes work to facilitate eudaimonia, the flourishing and actualization, of the storytelling students.

The ethics–leadership pairing that we will employ most frequently in the rest of this work is the pairing of ethics of care and servant leadership. It, like the virtue/trait pairing, is a fully natural one; both an ethics of care and servant leadership put humans and their growth first, and indeed make it the primary goal of organizational or ethical action. They, like Kantian or nonconsequential ethics, assert that people are always ends in themselves and cannot be used defensibly as means to an end. Care ethics and servant leadership go further, though, and center eudaimonia as the purpose of ethical and organizational action. For human flourishing to occur, though, meaningfulness must be as ubiquitous as water is for fish. Think back for a second to the section above about Viktor Frankl in the concentration camp. Meaning (i.e., his scholarship) gave Frankl purpose and energy to live; in the very same moment, when meaning vanished for one of Frankl's fellow inmates, life for him was no longer sustainable. Humans are buoyed, and their world is shaped, by meaning. But if humans can create meaning (and they can), then it is evident that humans can manipulate their own conditions for survival, and indeed, even their own flourishing. For meaning to operate, choice must be an integral part of that meaning. *Meaning* and *choice*, then, will also play central roles in our contemplations of heroism.

There is a very real danger in the idea that all truth is relative. It leads to the assertion of the possibility of "alternative facts" that can threaten the very fabric of meaningful discourse. Such a thing as alternative facts is not remotely what we intend when we indicate that there is relativity in some kinds of truth. More than merely affirming voices that have been marginalized, the celebration of multiple truths among humans actually works to create a fuller sense of wider Human Truth. Viewed correctly, then, the assertion of "alternative facts" does not validate the alternative facts themselves, but it does indicate the existence of a brand of human reality. This reality is a result of *suffering or affliction*, the very thing that heroes often find themselves confronting. We should pay close attention, then, to the nature of suffering or affliction.

The set of things we have identified here – capacities and potentialities, context, human flourishing, meaning and choice, and suffering/affliction – are by no means the only themes we could employ. They are the themes that for us seem most evident, probably in no small way because of our own contemplations. It is not our purpose here to list every conceivable aspect of heroism to be derived from thinking about normative ethics and leadership theory. Such a list would take more than one book, and in the end likely would be rather less value than one might assume. Instead, as we trace our argument from the theories above to the examples offered by students and our conclusions about them, we invite you to create your own argument from theory and your data, including your own experiences.

BOX 3.1 LEADERSHIP NOTES

An effective leader focuses on a more holistic, big picture, long-term view of effectiveness, as well as more short-term efficiency concerns. The old saying, "happy wife, happy life," may also in a way apply to those persons one leads. A workplace setting tends to be more efficient and more effective where a sense of meaning and purpose exists. Such a leader recognizes that the ends don't always justify the means in meeting a production goal or administrative objective. While, perhaps, it might take a bit longer, the "small way" of doing things often proves essential to accomplishing large goals. It is not enough to pay lip service to good intentions. Good intentions have to be *acted upon*. Simple acts of thoughtfulness and kindness build a reservoir of goodwill and trust within a working community. Such an approach is forward looking and person as well as product or results driven.

With virtue ethics, we come to understand that cultivating the communal good in both the communities we work and live in makes our life and those we work with more satisfying and meaningful. No matter what leadership style we prefer, we make choices and consequences follow. For every action, there is a reaction. If our actions are knowledge-based and we persevere in striving to do what is right as well as what works, we increase the chances that we will end up building character in ourselves, in our peers and in those we supervise. In both the formal and informal structure and process of organizations, where heroism and good leadership are concerned, one leads by example. And yes, sometimes, it seems too often, good isn't rewarded and the bad guys win. Still, it remains true: *the leader who possesses charisma without character is at her or his core a charlatan.*

Ethical leaders with a moral compass exude a different kind of charisma, perhaps at times, exuberant and on other occasions, lower-keyed. Such leaders have both a healthy emotional and an intellectual IQ. They demonstrate effective negotiation and diplomatic skills, creating wherever and whenever they can, win-win outcomes. Under the right circumstances, through their transactional effectiveness, such leaders can evolve into a kind of transformational example, creating a working context and environment where they and those they work with are creative and highly productive, even becoming more than they thought they could be.

Questions

1   What does being a "good person" mean to you? What about what constitutes being a good leader? In considering normative and virtue ethics, which approach appeals most to you? Why?

2   In thinking about normative and virtue ethics as well as utilitarian and deontological perspectives, how does our search for meaning square with our desire to do good, not just for ourselves, but for others as well?

3   Our personal character for better and worse comes from the quality of our lived-out values and moral beliefs. What values do you hold dear? Where did they come from? How would you like to translate and integrate into the work you commit yourself to?

References

Aristotle. (2019). *Nicomachean ethics*. Accessed May 19, 2019, 9:20pm from http://classics.mit.edu/Aristotle/nicomachaen.html

Barnard, C. (1938/1971). *The functions of the executive*. Boston, MA: Harvard University Press.

Bass, B., & Riggio, R. (2006). *Transformational leadership*. Mahwah, NJ: Lawrence Erlbaum & Assoc.

Blake, J., & Mouton, R. (1966). *The managerial grid: Leadership styles for achieving production through people*. Houston, TX: Gulf Publishing.

Boyatzis, R., & McKee, A. (2005). *Resonant leadership: Renewing yourself and connecting with others through mindfulness, hope and compassion*. Boston, MA: Harvard Business School.

Braswell, M. (2018). *The memory of grace*. Madison, WI: Borderland Books.

Braswell, M., McCarthy, B., & McCarthy, B. (eds.). (2020). *Justice, crime and ethics* (10th ed.). New York: Routledge.

Burns, J. (1978). *Leadership*. New York: Harper & Row.

Dahl, R. (1957). The concept of power. *Behavioral Science: Journal for the Society of General Systems Research 2*, 3, 201–215.

DeValve, M. (2007). *Purpose, power, justice and marginality: An examination of key prerequisites for diversity at the Texas Department of Criminal Justice*. Saarbrucken, Germany: VDM Verlag.

DeValve, M., Garland, T., & Wright, B. (2018). *A unified theory of justice and crime: Justice that love gives*. Lanham, MD: Lexington/Rowman & Littlefield.Fiedler, F. (2006). The contingency model: A theory of leadership effectiveness. In Levine, J., & Moreland, R. (eds.). *Small groups: Key readings*. Pp. 369–382. Hove: Psychology Press.

Frankl, V. (2006). *Man's search for meaning*. Boston, MA: Beacon.

Friedland, H. (2016). Navigating through narratives of despair: Making space for the Cree reasonable person in the Canadian justice system. *University of New Brunswick Law Journal 67*, 270–310.

Gardner, J. (2015). The many faces of the reasonable person. *Law Quarterly Review 131*, 563–584.

Gilligan, C. (1993). *In a different voice: Psychological theory and women's development*. Cambridge, MA: Harvard University Press.

Goleman, D. (2005). *Emotional intelligence: Why it can matter more than IQ*. New York: Bantam.

Greenleaf, R. (2003). The servant as leader (original 1970 edition). In Beazley, H., Beggs, J., & Spears, L. (eds.). *The servant-leader within: A transformative path*. New York and Mahwah, NJ: Paulist. Pp. 29–74.

Hersey, P., & Blanchard, K. (1969). *Management of organizational behavior: Utilizing human resources*. Upper Saddle River, NJ: Prentice-Hall.

Hofstede, G. (1991). *Cultures and organizations: Software of the mind*. New York: McGraw-Hill.

House, R., & Mitchell, T. (1975). *Path-goal theory of leadership*. Office of Naval Research Report. Washington, DC: NTIS, U.S. Department of Commerce.

Kahn, R., & Katz, D. (1968). Leadership practices in relation to productivity and morale. In Cartwright, D., & Zander, A. (eds.). *Group dynamics: Research and theory, (3d)*. New York: Harper & Row. Pp. 362–380.

Kleingeld, P. (2019). A contradiction of the right kind: Convenience killing and Kant's formula of universal law. *The Philosophical Quarterly 69*, 274, 64–81.

Levin, M. (1997). Natural subordination, Aristotle on. *Philosophy 72*, 280, 241–257.

Lewin, K., Lippitt, R., & White, R. (1939). Patterns of aggressive behavior in experimentally created "social climates." *Journal of Social Psychology 10*, 271–299.

Liebeck v. McDonald's Restaurants, 1994 extra LEXIS 23; Bernalillo Co. N.M. Dist, Ct. 1994.

Likert, R. (1967). *The human organization: Its management and value*. New York: McGraw-Hill.

Maslow, A. (1943). A theory of human motivation. *Psychological Review 50*, 1, 370–396.

Osborne, D., & Gaebler, T. (1992). *Reinventing government: How the entrepreneurial spirit is transforming the public sector.* New York: Plume/Penguin.

Phair, D. (2017). Searching for the appropriate standard: Stops, seizures, and the reasonable person's willingness to walk away from the police. *Washington Law Review 92,* 1, 425–479.

Senge, P. (2006). *The fifth discipline: The art and practice of the learning organization.* New York: Doubleday.

Taylor, F. (2014). *The principles of scientific management.* Eastford, CT: Martino Fine Books.

Terry v. Ohio, 392 U.S. 1. (1968).

Tichy, N., & Devanna, M. (1997). *The transformational leader: The key to global competitiveness.* Hoboken, NJ: John Wiley and Sons.

United States v. Carroll Towing Co., 159 F2d at 169. (1947).

Vitiello, M. (2010). Defining the reasonable person in the criminal law: Fighting the Lernaean hydra. *Lewis & Clark Law Review 14,* 4, 1435–1454.

Weil, S. (2015a). What is sacred in every human being? In Weil, S. (eds.). *Simone Weil: Late philosophical writings.* Springstead, E. (trans.). Notre Dame, IN: University of Notre Dame Press. Pp. 103–129.

Weil, S. (2015b). Essay on the concept of reading. In Weil, S. (eds.). *Simone Weil: Late philosophical writings.* Springstead, E. (trans.). Notre Dame, IN: University of Notre Dame Press. Pp. 21–28.

Wren, D. (2005). *The history of management thought* (5th ed.). Hoboken, NJ: John Wiley and Sons.

4

THE MAKING OF A HERO

Responding to Life's Challenges and the Needs of Others

Along with an entourage of nearly 100 people and their accoutrement, including everything from imported British limestone markers to a featherbed-nested telescope, two men set off into the American wilderness in order to settle a dispute. Jeremiah Dixon and Charles Mason had been recruited from among the most well regarded of their professions (surveyor and astronomer, respectively) and given the charge of drawing the line between the colonies of Maryland and Pennsylvania, over which more than a little wrangling had occurred. They set out into a land full of threats and almost totally absent of guarantees. As it turns out, they achieved a level of precision that is praiseworthy by even today's standards.

What has become known as the Mason-Dixon Line was intended to settle tax disputes between just the two colonies, now states, it divides, but it has become emblematic of both unconscionable violence and the promise of freedom. When the two men and their team left Philadelphia in 1763, though, there was nothing like certainty regarding its completion or precision, let alone the deep cultural significance it would take on in later years. The Mason-Dixon Line, which has come to mean so many things in American culture, began with little more than a collection of materiel, the dedication of a few stalwart experts and their charge of responsibility. It is fair to say that Mason and Dixon did a truly heroic thing, that they're heroes. What they accomplished has been likened to the *Apollo* moon landings for their time. It was not an expedition into *herodom* that they undertook. They did not anticipate praise or high office, only challenges; many unknown, some potentially lethal. The key point here, though, is that they were not heroes until they were.

The cliché that hindsight is 20-20 has more than a little wisdom to it in point of fact. With the benefit of time one can view past moments through the lens of a kind of revelation; knowing what the future holds can seem to wring insight and meaning from past circumstances and events, giving them a contour and content that was not present, at the least not evident, in the moment. It might seem, looking back, as if the present state of affairs is already etched indelibly upon the past somehow. Aside from the senior discount at Sizzler or other restaurants, one of the most fertile benefits of getting older is the trunk full of experiences one has gathered over time. Often, if one does the job of getting older correctly, those experiences are faceted and polished such that they channel light in ways that make life more meaningful and just a little easier.

The idea of nonduality posits that we as human beings are individually viable organisms. We are not fused to each other, nor are we inextricably rooted to the ground like trees. At the same time, nonduality asserts that we are fully dependent upon others and upon the world around us, even in ways indistinguishable from them. We are *earthen* beings, *of* this place as much as *from* this place. We are distinct and yet we belong to each other. We are individuals and we are fully interdependent in both apparent and hidden ways.

This nonduality applies just as richly to how we as sentient, thinking, feeling, creating beings think, feel and create. Our *state* of being *is* the *process* of becoming. Being is becoming and becoming is being. This insight has at least two consequences in relation to heroes and heroism. First, it means that the process of becoming a hero is not distinct from *simply being.* We might perceive from this that heroism is not so much a thing toward which one strives actively but is more a thing into which one stumbles and falls backward. Heroism is not planned as much as it is dictated or activated by circumstance, which is why we hear it said of heroes, "heroes rise to the occasion."

Second, and possibly more significant, is that the potential hero exists as hero, fully fledged, even before any heroic event sealed the deal. There is something else, though. When we call someone "heroic" or perceive "heroism" in another, it necessarily means that aspects of the hero also live in "us," the one who places the "hero" label on another person or action.

Think again of Achilles: champion, yes, but hardly the hero for which we might hope. Think also of Galahad as he ascended to heaven, Grail in hand. He isn't exactly the hero we want when we call 911. Genuine heroes do not set out to be heroes and for this reason perhaps more than any other, they become heroes. At the same time, there is something of the hero discernible in the water-bearer before the title "hero" fully can be given.

And speaking of becoming heroes, it is time for our attention to turn to the stars of the show: the students and their heroes. Much of the rest of this book will be given over to the contemplation of what students have said about their everyday, ordinary heroes.

In this first chapter to feature students and their heroes, somewhat naturally we begin with a contemplation of the making of heroes – by what process heroes come to be heroes. And a good bit of what comes next, though organized by us, is in the voices of students themselves. In terms of the organization, with regard to how heroes respond to life's challenges and others' needs, we have identified four themes emerging from students' writings, and a fifth overarching theme: being and becoming. These four themes are inclusiveness, loyalty, courage and humility.

Now, let us be clear: it is not our contention that if we take these four attributes coupled with the overarching theme and added them to some kind of blender that heroism would come out the other side. Of course, heroes and heroism are not baked goods: we don't combine ingredients according to recipe and come out with a scone called heroism. In their experiences, though, students pointed to attributes they perceived as constitutive capacities – attributes they perceive in the people they held up as heroes that seemed significant to them as they understood the process of hero-becoming. In this, these four attributes – inclusiveness, loyalty, courage and humility – were things commonly perceived among students regarding their heroes in terms of "how" their heroes became heroes.

Let us turn to a closer examination of each of these four themes, holding in mind the grand theme of being and becoming. And one more thing: although we will use names in our recounting of students' statements, all names are pseudonyms.

Inclusiveness

Achilles, if you recall, raged against the walls of Troy. Others have stood on walls against besieging armies for millennia since Troy's walls tumbled into dust. In the eyes of students, though, walls, at least metaphorical ones, were razed by heroes and bridges made in their place. In this we should not think so much in terms of Joshua sounding trumpets to level Jericho's defenses, but in terms of making a way smooth, of dozing rocky terrain to make something possible and passable. Heroes become heroes through uniting people with people, and people with their own capacities, their own potentialities, and students made this clear.

Sam and Gabriel

"Sam" writes about his best friend's twin brothers with cerebral palsy. One of the two, "Gabriel," is the hero about whom he writes. Gabriel can get around with the aid of a walker, but when Gabriel is about town, people he meets are often anxious to help him, say, open a door. The sight of someone in a wheelchair or behind a walker seems often to trigger helping behavior. Such unexamined helping behavior is not itself necessarily problematic, of course, but it does not come without something of a cost. In many instances, it is both accommodating and appreciated when someone holds the door open for someone else. Yet, for someone like Gabriel, such an action could have a different effect. According to his mother, Gabriel wanted very much to be seen as "normal." Offering to help without some measure of contemplation can create its own kind of hardship. The offer to hold a door open often comes when the need for help seems obvious, and that obviousness can be a kind of prison for the one the help is intended for. At least that might be the sense one has being in Gabriel's circumstance.

Clearly, "normal" has a very clear meaning to Gabriel, one that might be tricky for many of us to put a finger on. It is tempting for us at this considerable remove to take Gabriel's meaning of normalcy to be about opening his own doors without help or fanfare. Sam does not elaborate on the daily circumstances in which Gabriel lives, but he does give us a sense of one rather particular way in which Gabriel is not only normal but also heroic. Gabriel, it seems, maintains a robust sense of humor. The challenges before him are not easily countable by us; to maintain a smile and joke about one's hardships is a truly remarkable capacity. His humor in the face of hardship taught Sam that nothing is insurmountable. It seems that Gabriel, in no small way because of his humor, not only lives richly but also empowers others to smile while sharing his challenges and facing their own.

What is really telling about Sam's and Gabriel's story, though, is that Sam is in many ways also the hero in his story about Gabriel the Hero. Sam came to understand at a deeper level that Gabriel sought only to be "normal." Sam accepted Gabriel's understanding of normalcy on Gabriel's terms. As children growing up together, they joked and played games together without a sense of difference or awkwardness. Sam knew Gabriel because he experienced and knew him in a very deep way. Further, he loved Gabriel by honoring in big ways and small his need for normalcy as he conceived it.

Humility

One of the more counterintuitive things about heroism is that truest heroism is not a thing toward which one aims one's life energy. While still quite young, the daughter of one of the authors informed her parental committee that she intended to become an entomologist when she grew up. This is a slightly odd thing for a five-year-old to assert, perhaps, but quite a bit odder would be if the same child had informed her parental committee that she had decided to become a hero when she grew up.

But wait: is it not the case that at some fundamental level, we as sentient beings seek to be relevant to others of our species, to the point of being remembered after we have ceased to be? It is, we think, an interesting exercise to contemplate precisely how long after death and for what we would seek to be remembered. If even some of us have a deep drive to be relevant after we return to dust, why *not* strive to be a hero?

In fairness, if Aristotle was on to something, we might well conclude that if the (or one) purpose of parenting and public education is the cultivation of practical reason (phronesis), then it is reasonable to argue that parenting and education are organized human activities that strive to create *potential* heroes: parenting and education strive to make people who are ready to rise to an occasion but were just missing an occasion.

But all of this misses a crucial element in what we understand today to be heroism. Heroes – truest heroes – do not seek such status and may even have sought to avoid it. Arthur was not out and about looking for metaphysical anointment for his designs on leadership. Claudette Colvin, perhaps the clearest example from earlier, had been exposed to the examples of Sojourner Truth and Harriet Tubman; essentially, her practical reason had been cultivated. Given the choice between segregation never having been and her having the moment align for her to become a hero, it seems likely she would have chosen the former. It seems reasonable to assume Dr. King would have preferred to have died quietly in his bed of old age after a lifetime of humble and quiet service to his congregation. Heroes, at least the heroes that seem to compel us most today, would prefer to have nothing to do with heroism.

When the occasion arises, though, heroes do indeed rise. Heroes do hard things, things that need to be done, often when others cannot or will not do those things. Heroes seem to have a refined sense of when to stand in front and take risks for others and when to stand back and let others receive acclaim.

And of course, this is the case. It is in the very nature of heroism as we seem to understand it to put others before self even (and especially) when that means stepping forward. Were one to celebrate one's own act of selflessness in a fashion akin to an NFL wide receiver scoring a touchdown, we would be more than a little off-putting. No, whether for standing up or drifting back, the title "hero" is a thing conferred most meaningfully when the person receiving the title is least likely to ratify it.

Jeanne and Her Dad

It is only natural, Jeanne tells us, for a daughter to admire her father. For her, though, her admiration grew immensely when she learned more about her father's life as a young man. He was the only boy in a big farming family, named after his grandfather. His circumstances were both idyllic and constrained: the land was bountiful, and the living was stark and clean. It was clear, though, that he was the hope for the future of the farm. From one perspective, the choices many of us enjoy regarding what we will do with our lives were made already for Jeanne's dad; the expectation was that he would take over the farm.

But choice is a funny thing. Even when we feel as if we have no choice whatsoever, we have a choice regarding how we confront our choice-lessness, and so regain our choice. Jeanne's dad had had broad and weighty expectations placed upon him at a young age. Then fate intervened. Back when Jeanne's dad was still in high school, an impolitic mule kicked Jeanne's dad's dad solidly enough to break his femur. Such an injury would lay anyone low for a time, and this was the case for Jeanne's dad's dad. The farm needed tending, though; the animals and crops would not wait for a bone to heal. Jeanne's dad decided to end his education and to take up carrying the farm himself. In every family there are moments: moments that define, moments that shape the future. Jeanne swells when she talks about how the family responded when Jeanne's dad chose the farm, essentially over himself.

There's something else Jeanne tells us about her dad that bears considering here. One might think that someone given over to clawing a living from the soil would see the world in terms of a work ethic: what one gets is a result of what one has done. You don't eat if you don't work. That's not how Jeanne's dad operates. Indeed, the very opposite is the case. His generosity, particularly toward families who have little, is remarkable. One of his favorite strategies for confronting need, Jeanne tells us, is to organize fundraising pig roasts.

Jeanne's grandfather's femur has long since healed, and Jeanne's dad has made another choice. In fairness, he makes many choices every day, though in the final analysis it is the very same choice he has made all along: the choice to serve humbly.

Andrew's Great-Uncle

Ever seeming to seek validation, the noise we make in search of interaction and approval proliferates, reverberates. Significant silence seems increasingly rare. Sometimes it seems that people today are more inclined than ever to talk rather than listen. Then there's that person – perhaps you know someone like this – who rests in silence like a warm sea. When that person speaks, people listen. Andrew's great-uncle was just such a person.

Often those who experience the horrors of war testify to the unspeakableness of their experience by their silence. For those of us who can only wonder about what they went through, we can only speculate as to the nature of their silence and the interior world to which it points; some may seek to strategize the use of their voice so that they can be more effective when it counts. Some others are cowed by experience and can only offer silence. Neither seems to be the case for Andrew's great-uncle. Instead, Andrew's great-uncle is unassuming, but his unassuming nature cuts a larger-than-life figure in Andrew's memory.

It was a beautiful Sunday morning, we are told, typical for early December mornings in Hawaii. Andrew's great-uncle tells of having seen shark fins in the harbor on previous occasions, but something seemed different about the one he saw this morning. It was only when the shark was 25 feet from him that he realized it was not a shark at all. The torpedo seems to have missed the boat on which he stood, but the story of the Japanese attack on Pearl Harbor is well known in gory detail. That's all we know, though, about Andrew's great-uncle's experience, because that is all Andrew was ever told. A dignified silence, befitting the silence of the USS *Arizona*, is what remains. It is the silence that comes because there is nothing that could ever be said.

Andrew's great-uncle operated from a mighty silence, but not always was it the silence of a tomb. It was a strong but unassuming silence, not a silence that comes from seeking to be significant. It was the kind of humility that draws attention, the kind of unassumingness that begs trust. Andrew tells us that he did not have the chance to get to know his great-uncle the way he would have liked; the occasional family gathering was the setting for most of their interactions. The silence authored by Andrew's great-uncle seems to have had a far more profound impact on Andrew than volumes ever could.

Kevin's Grandfather

The church is silent but for the sibilance of the wheels on the padded carpet and a faint mechanical squeak of the poorly greased axle. The man in the chair is old and clearly infirm, missing one leg up to the hip. He is dressed in an old suit coat, tired tie and button-up shirt. The empty pant leg is folded carefully beneath the stump that once bore his frame. His son pushes the chair to the front of the church, pauses pridefully behind him and then sits. And as the old man breathes in to speak, the congregation breathes in time with him, for him.

It is easy to give thanks when life is good, when you have your health. It is a different matter altogether to give thanks when there is no clear future, when your body is systematically disassembled by a disease while you watch. Kevin's hero is his grandfather. Kevin's grandfather had diabetes and a heart condition. As his disease state worsened, his kidneys failed, tying him to dialysis. Eventually, poor circulation claimed his leg. The wound never healed, however, so he was unable to use prostheses. Wheelchair-bound, he continued to weaken over the last months. Never in any of this, though, did Kevin's grandfather cease to give thanks or lose himself to his own misery. He praised, not only in word but also in deed, thinking of others before himself. His loving kindness was not a function of privilege or wellbeing; he did not give from a position of having and his hope came not from a place of expectancy. He focused on others when his own circumstance was clearly dire.

Helen's Mom

Even among heroes there are some who are, well, extraordinary. Helen's mom is one of those heroes. Helen and her family emigrated from a country south of the United States. While there, Helen's mother fashioned a home of their own for the family from adobe with her own hands. Helen tells us how she recalls seeing her mother digging ditches to make adobe. The family sought a more prosperous life for their children, so they emigrated to the United States. Life was not easier, however, at least for Helen's mom. Although she was not forced to build the family's home, Helen's mom worked a demanding job at a factory. She worked long, taxing hours, often coming home weeping from the pain in her swollen arms. She developed tendinitis, arthritis and a slipped disc in her back. Helen's mom often skipped meals so that her children had enough to eat. Helen's mom quite literally ground her own body down to a nub for her family.

Helen's mom did all she did not only so that her children could eat, but also so that they would not have to live as she has lived. Helen's mom learned many hard lessons and she was anxious to impart those lessons to her children, sometimes through her own bodily sacrifice. Helen speaks about how her mom emphasized the value of education. At the same time, Helen's mom forbade Helen from looking down on those who do not have an education, forbade her to forget where she came from. Finally, she taught Helen not to be reliant upon a man, to be her own woman.

Helen's mom counseled humility despite capacity. What is rather more compelling, though, is that she lived humility: she did jobs that literally broke her body, jobs that were menial and thankless. She dug ditches, making herself literally low in order to elevate those she loved. Thankless, menial, bone-snapping work undertaken for another for the sake of love: a powerfully moving example of humility in heroism.

Loyalty

The term "loyalty" might be a little confusing, at least at the outset. After all, being loyal to a person can rather quickly turn from heroic into something quite a bit less noble. Being loyal to someone can be decidedly unheroic, in fact. At the same time, loyalty can be fiercely heroic at times. How, then, are we to understand loyalty in the context of becoming a hero?

Think back to our conversation in the previous chapter regarding ethics. We said that heroism often and almost by definition goes above and beyond most normative ethical systems by acting in super-ethical ways. It is precisely the fact that an action, like putting others before yourself at your own considerable risk or expense, is not expected or called for by an ethical system that makes it heroic. In a sense, then, a hero authors her own superordinate ethical system through her action. What is more, though, is that they stick to that system, in idea and action. They are loyal to their own super-ethical conception of how to act and think. They are consistently doing heroic things that are, again, by definition, beyond expectation. They live up to promises made by past idea and action; they can today cash the checks they write with deeds and words of the past. They keep their promises. And all of it, the action and words of the past and those of today all point to heroic ideas like those we have discussed so far (selflessness, other-actualization and the rest).

Part of the consistency of heroes, their tendency to do heroic things repeatedly, is that they are not doing heroism as such: they are not typically setting out to be heroic but merely to "do what was called for," or "do what is right" in a given circumstance. We saw already how this tendency for heroes to become heroes precisely by not aiming to be heroes in the first place tends to operate, but here it is our interest to highlight the idea of *consistent* heroism; truest heroes are not fair-weather affairs. Heroism is not heroism, reframing Shakespeare's famous words, "which alters when it alteration finds." Heroism is "an ever fixed mark" that cannot see itself in such terms. If there is a planet that orbits the cool sun Polaris, and if there are sentient occupants that dwell there, that their home star has played such a profoundly significant role in the lives of countless occupants of this planet, guiding them to safety, to feeding grounds, or home to loved ones, may well matter little.

Gary's Mom and Walter Payton

Another one of those extraordinary heroes among heroes would be Gary's mom. She raised Gary from a young age by herself, which would be feat enough. She also put herself through nursing school while supporting their small family. Gary's mom repeatedly has gone without food so that others had enough to eat. Despite all of this, Gary's mom is the most giving and caring person he knows. Instead of being hardened by hardship, she has stubbornly insisted on being loving.

Gary also indicates that Walter Payton, the former running back for the Chicago Bears, is his hero. Payton, he says, was the finest running back to play the game, but that he never acted as if this were the case. He did not make a show or become corrupted by the money he received. He played, Gary says, because he loved the game, not because he craved the limelight. He played for a team that enjoyed few successes (although they won the Super Bowl in Payton's last year before retirement) but did not complain. He did not seek to leverage his impressive statistics to make more money or to trade to a more prosperous team. He stuck with his team through thick and thin, not because they paid him, but because he believed it was the right thing to do.

Gary asserts that his two heroes had little in common, but we disagree. Both Gary's mom and Walter Payton represent a kind of constancy, an adherence to principle despite consequences, that is remarkable. Gary's mom lives her commitment to nurturance. Nursing school is no cakewalk. She chose to nurture him while learning to nurture others, so that she could make a better living with which to nurture him, while actualizing (nurturing) herself by furthering her education. She showed Gary how important education was by prioritizing her own education. Had she earned a degree in *anything*, the point would have been made, but as it turns out, she studied *nursing*; the point, then, could not be clearer: in every aspect of her life she chose nurturance. Walter Payton also practiced and modeled a sense of constancy in values. Hailed as one of the finest running backs in the NFL, he nonetheless played for what was for years one of the weakest teams in the league. He could have left Chicago no doubt, and for quite a bit more money, but he did not, because he would not. That his loyalty was repaid poetically and in spades in the body of the 1985–1986 Bears, who proceeded to trounce most comers and to win the Super Bowl that season in *decisive* fashion, could not have been foreseen.

Lori's Family

Often a child born to a 14-year-old mom begins at a stark disadvantage. Lori was different, however, for several reasons: the members of her immediate family. Her mom was to prove herself exceptional, of course, raising Lori and providing for her while attending school, but Lori's mom was far from alone. Lori's uncle ended his own schooling so that Lori would have someone at home. Lori's grandmother, great-grandmother and great-great-uncle all lived with her and each played a significant role in her growth into the woman she became.

Lori's great-grandmother repeatedly cautioned Lori about boys: boys are "low-down" and not to be trusted. She also introduced Lori to church and thus to singing. Lori's grandmother taught her "girly" things: hair, makeup and such. Lori's uncle taught her to cook and how to use a computer; he and she were very close through much of her childhood.

In Lori's life, each of the several members of her immediate family contributed to her actualization. Lori's mother found herself in a profoundly difficult place very early in life, but instead of isolating her, the family gathered around Lori and her mother. In adversity, the family fused and, in so doing, succeeded in elevating all. She describes her family as "small but loyal"; indeed so.

Courage

Aristotle would not be, well, Aristotle, if he did not swat a few home runs. One of those home runs is the idea of courage: As we indicated earlier, being courageous is not being without fear. Quite the opposite is the case, in fact: courage *presupposes* fear. Without fear, courage is hollow; it isn't courage, at least it is not heroic.

Robert and His Grandfather

Nonduality means that it can be tricky determining specifically where heroism resides. Is heroism a thing that happens in the moment and is fully recognized as such, or is heroism only heroism with the benefit of hindsight? Both might well be true, and for different circumstances, of course. "Robert" told us about his grandfather just now. Robert's grandfather did many things, none of which was for him heroic but, in the end, were indeed heroic in the eyes of his grandson. We know scarce little about his service as a teacher and principal, and nothing at all about his experiences during the war. What we do know, though, is how people remembered him to Robert: he was one who did for others without thought of return, again and again, and as one who practiced a lifelong commitment to actualizing others.

The things he did, though, from his experiences in the war and fighting for racial equality in education to the tiny efforts on behalf of others required of him to make a stand despite being afraid of what that stand could become. It is likely that he faced death in combat, and it is also likely that he faced entrenched enemies in his efforts to desegregate his schools. It would be insane not to have been afraid in either of these circumstances. The point, though, is that Robert's grandfather did the hard things with which he had been tasked despite the fear he felt.

Timmy's Brother

It would be difficult to imagine a more nightmarish scenario: your family is directly in the path of an army of drug-fueled child-soldiers roaming the countryside killing, raping and maiming at will. Timmy and his family found themselves in this very circumstance in 1990. Nearly a quarter of a million people were killed and many more were maimed and injured during the first Liberian Civil War. Charles Taylor and his National Patriotic Front of Liberia authored a symphony of sickening brutality in Liberia for nearly seven years, the likes of which have few analogs in human history.

The family sought some measure of safety by fleeing to nearby Ghana. The refugee camp in which they lived, though, was only marginally safer than war-torn Liberia was: clean food and water were scarce and shelter was truly meager. Death form illness and exposure was a constant in the camp. The United Nations intervened to provide safer food and water, but conditions in the camp were only barely tolerable. Something had to be done.

In 1998, Timmy's brother entered the Diversity Immigrant Visa lottery in the hope of securing some exit for the family. He won, but winning the lottery was the easiest part of the ordeal. He had to purchase his own air fare and, once there, provide for himself. Well, Timmy's brother succeeded. After a time in the United States by himself, he earned his citizenship, and then sent for his family to join him. Timmy, former resident of a Liberian refugee camp, with no clear hope of healthy food, water or shelter, let alone an actualizing education, told us about his hero from the opportunity-rich seat in an American university classroom.

To be sure, desperation compels extraordinary action, but consider for a moment what it must have been like for Timmy's brother: in order to rescue your family from crushing deprivation and possible death, you must move to a wholly unfamiliar place, one known for grinding dreams into dust. You have no resources, no safe landing place and no support network, and in this unfamiliar free-market Mecca you must find a place to live, the legal means to pay bills, and you must amass enough of a "nest-egg" to secure passage for your family to join you. The pressure on him must have been extraordinary indeed, and the courage required to face the thousand unforeseen challenges, not to mention the foreseeable ones, is most certainly worthy of the highest admiration.

Marius' Dad

It is an extraordinary thing to know who and what you want to be, and then to become that thing, when your family is vehemently and actively opposed to your becoming that thing. Marius tells us about his dad. Marius' dad and his two sisters grew up in a low-wealth, single-parent home. Mom was constantly working in order to provide for the children, so the children were on their own much of the time. Marius' dad concluded that education was his path out of poverty and deprivation. He excelled in school through both natural ability and tireless effort.

Where things became problematic for Marius' dad is with regard to his particular aspirations. His grades in school earned him admission to The Citadel. His family, however, was deeply opposed to a military career for him, to the point where their relationship is estranged even today. Marius' dad became an officer in the U.S. military and has since retired as a colonel after a distinguished career in military intelligence. Marius' dad chose the military for a career despite every influence his family – undoubtedly a close family for its shared suffering – could render. It took courage to know himself well enough to see the shape of his dreams; it took even more courage to confront his family with the shape of his dreams. It took yet more courage to choose to follow his dreams despite what it might, and indeed has, cost him.

Conclusion

Heroes become, and yet heroes are already. The ordeals that constitute the raw material of heroism are themselves the very last thing from heroism as such. They are difficult, often ugly and almost always dangerous in some way. In the becoming, heroism is not heroism. At the same time, there is something profoundly beautiful, something evidently heroic, in the hero that has been there all the time. That sounds like a contradiction, but the truth of it sits in high relief in the stories we have heard.

Perhaps we might understand it this way: the acts that give meaning to the moniker "hero" or "heroism" are themselves not glorious acts, and neither are they undertaken for the sake of earning the title. They are ugly, dangerous, uncertain, often thankless. There are foreseen and unforeseen challenges, each carrying their own burdens. None of them, and none of them taken together, could be meaningfully called heroism. Only in the larger context of why they were undertaken does the label "heroism" make sense. And that leads us to the other point.

What makes the digging of a ditch to make an adobe house heroism is why it was undertaken: love. What makes clawing a living from the soil or wresting it from machines in a factory heroism is why it is done: love. Desegregating a school system, teaching a child how to make pasta, sticking with a losing team and alienating one's sisters have much in common when context of the acts is considered. These are acts of heroism because of the human truth they serve.

Charles Mason and Jeremiah Dixon strode into the wilds before them and into an uncertain future. The task was to trace a path through uncertainty for the benefit of many thousands of people, most of whom they would never meet. Progress took the form of distance covered; each mile was commemorated with a limestone marker situated with the sides marked "P" and "M" facing the proper directions. They did not undertake the task of heroism as such. What might be heroism for us was for them a painstaking task of measuring, remeasuring and then situating stones, all in the context of the constant potential for lethal danger.

Consider Timmy's brother in this light: he had a mightily difficult set of tasks before himself, placed there by dark necessity. He constantly faced the prospect of catastrophic failure. All the while he could only hope for the best for his family in a UN refugee camp. Marius' dad might not have faced the same kind of desperation, but his challenge was no less poignant, his outcome no more certain. Andrew's great-uncle faced uncertainty in the body of a torpedo just barely missing him. How many more moments of hero-becoming he faced, we simply have no way of knowing.

BOX 4.1 LEADERSHIP NOTES

As one ascends the ladder of management success, the rungs of the ladder become narrower, the air gets thinner and the lack of oxygen can easily enough come to distort one's priorities and perceptions of reality. With fewer at the top of the career ladder, the people below can come to look smaller and less significant. Leaders who succumb to such a view engender an aura of exclusiveness, reinforcing each other's sense of expertise, more likely imagined than real. The old saying that we tend to "meet the same folks on the way down the ladder that we passed on the way up" often holds true.

An effective leader, one who can be heroic when a challenge emerges encourages similar qualities in those she or he supervises, embodying a kind of clear-eyed inclusiveness that exemplifies a collective "we are all in this together" mind-set. One of us, when beginning a semester's ethics class, would tell his students that while he might be the student in charge, the more important reality was that all who were part of the learning community were students, including himself. The main point was that all had something to contribute and learn from through the exchange of ideas.

Three essential qualities in the making of a leadership hero are humility, courage and loyalty. Humility is the starting point for the leader who is a hero in waiting. As we get older, as we become increasingly aware that we don't know all the answers or even all the questions, we find that we no longer have to "pretend" that we do. More mindful of our missteps and mistakes, we can become more open to what others have to say and, in turn, become more discerning in our decision-making. Rather exhibiting bluster, self-promotion and blaming others, we become more interested in seeing a problem solved than receiving the credit. Becoming more humble also leads us toward more courageous leadership choices. Instead of focusing on the end justifying the means with little or no regard for ethical ramifications, we strive to do what is right, to put our good intentions into action, to create win-win outcomes whenever possible.

Humble, courageous leaders cultivate loyalty from their peers and those persons they supervise. They don't sacrifice their humanity and integrity on the altar of short-term gain or success. Interestingly enough, insecure, self-absorbed leaders are just the opposite. They attempt to enforce loyalty through fear and intimidation, rewarding those who inflate their egos and feed their insatiable appetite for attention. They demand loyalty from others that they are incapable or unwilling to offer in return.

The hero-in-training maintains a beginner's mind more than an expert's whimsy, open and aware to what others have to offer. They are willing to take a chance to make a positive difference even when the outcome is uncertain. They embrace the challenge that is before them. They generously share the success with others when a victory is won and perhaps, more importantly, take responsibility and shoulder the blame when the collective effort results in failure.

Questions

1 How do you feel heroes are made? In considering student comments about the ordinary heroes that intervened in their lives, what do you think are the reasons some people step forward to meet the needs of another person while others choose to walk on by in one way or another?

2 Concerning the qualities of courage, loyalty and humility, which one do you believe is most important in the making of a hero? Why?

3 Why is cultivating and maintaining a "beginner's mind" important in responding to life's challenges and the needs of others?

5

HEROES AROUND US

A rose, Shakespeare tells us, would be just as perfumed were we to call it by any other name. And so it is with heroes; the beauty and goodness of their actions are, perhaps, just as praiseworthy, whether or not we call them "hero" or call what they do "heroism." For that matter, whether she is "mom," "Aunt Sally," "the biscuit lady," or "hey, you" might not matter at all. Heroism is just as powerful, just as exquisite from a parent as it is from a stranger.

There is something in the nature of some offices, though, some titles that lend themselves to heroism as we mean it here. At the same time, if title dictates heroism as a duty of office, it probably isn't heroism in the fullest sense after all is said and done (although there may be some notable exceptions). Again, heroism seems almost to necessitate that heroic action is a thing that operates clearly and above duty and expectation. Central to heroism is choice: the choice to act, to serve, to become involved, to love enough to risk failure or, in some instances, even one's life. Choice matters not only in terms of whether to act, but also how to act, and even determining what successful action might look like.

It would not serve as well as one might think, then, to think first, about the roles heroes play in the lives of the students who speak through this work, and then to think about the nature of their heroes' courageous acts. In other words, we will not examine the heroism of moms as such, in comparison to the heroism of siblings, friends or strangers. If title dictated behavior, heroism as we understand it would change radically. It would be expected from certain people (e.g., moms) but not from others. Moms would always leap into the lion's den to protect their children. In fact, it would be weird if a mom failed to do the exceptional thing. And if we really look at the nature of the human condition, we would always choose to save each other, in great moments and small, in every chance presented to us. Moments of heroic grace would be normalized.

If title can't matter all that much, then why contemplate office at all? We contemplate it because it *does* seem to matter, at least somewhat. Title, responsibility, circumstance and choice are not related in a simple linear fashion, but title does indeed seem to be relevant to our understanding of heroism. It would not be a surprise, for example, to read about a mom leaping into danger to rescue her toddler son who had fallen through the thin icy crust and into the frigid water. Learning that a police officer had done the same thing might surprise us only slightly more. A *stranger*, though…, now that's a different story…, perhaps. Title or office seems to be related somehow to the topography of expectations for the potential hero as viewed by the potential beneficiary of heroism. The same holds true for the wider community, and by the potential hero her- or himself, but title is in no way a sufficient indicator of heroism or the establishment of heroes.

It is tempting to assume heroism is partly a result of a utilitarian calculus: those who are more compelled to jump into heroism may be those with the most to lose. Moms, for instance: something dies in a mother along with her child when she buries him or her. Such a view fails us, though, in that it portrays us as rational, benefit-ruled beings with only a weak-tea emotional existence. Nothing could be further from the truth. Regardless of title, incentives don't a hero make.

What, then, is the nature of the relationship between title or responsibility and our understanding of heroism? In this chapter we will examine heroism through our students' insights in terms of the identities of those they hold up as heroes. We do this in order to direct our focus. Title may not create heroism, but it is fair to think that title might in some way shape heroism. How and to what degree will be the thing we pursue in this chapter.

Family

Such a thing as this can never be repeated too often: we, the authors of this book, wish to say to our families that anything we ever do of value is in one way or another because of them. Parents, spouses, aunts and uncles, cousins, children; this and all things are because of you. And how could it be otherwise, after all, when so much of what we are is a direct result of the selfless and unconditional investment in us made by people in our families?

Not everyone is so fortunate, having to raise themselves or their siblings without support, in a world of dark shadows and strange happenings, as a child trying to be a parent. For some, they have to somehow become their own hero through a kind of stubborn resistance to the neglect and abuse they are born into. And to be sure, even in the best of worlds, not every brother saves his sister's heart from implosion and not every mom finds herself working two jobs or having to dig ditches to make a home for her family. It is here that we find some of the real magic of choice to which these students bear witness; choices made, in this section, by those who love them most directly.

An Ode to Moms

It might surprise no one that almost one student in three named a mom (or grandmother) as the hero about which he or she wanted to write. The details often are truly humbling and deeply inspiring. We already met Helen's mom who dug ditches to make a home for her family and then quite literally broke her body on a factory wheel so her children could experience more serene and well-appointed lives. We also met Gary's mom, who routinely went without proper nutrition so her child could eat. Speaking to a point we made in the introduction, if we thought that office did not matter at all, we would be surprised to hear about the depth of the sacrifice made by Helen's or Gary's moms, but of course, we weren't. Still, not every mom would choose to cast herself into the flames so her children can enjoy a more hopeful life. The scale of sacrifice moms typically offer those for whom they care often coincides with the expectations we have for moms (and moms have for themselves). Such expectations tend to be greater than they are in other social role contexts. In other words, moms might act in more heroic ways, but we are also inclined to expect more, and more self-sacrifice from them. Let's turn to some moms in action.

Pat's Mom: A Mighty Oak

Consider the task: you are caring for your mentally ill mother when she is diagnosed with cancer. While supporting your family financially, you take time away from them to care for your mother through the course of her illness. Your mother's death is both crushing and something of a relief. A matter of *days* later, your sister is diagnosed with cancer, and a significant portion of her care falls on you. A matter of *days after that,* your sister's husband is murdered. Thich Nhat Hanh (e.g., 1975) talks about how we can seek to be like the trunk of a tree in the middle of a tempest; branches are tossed and torn about while the center holds and remains calm and unmoved. This is what was asked of Pat's mom. Anyone who has been through a hurricane knows, though, that every tree has its breaking point: a mighty oak can be felled when the winds are just that little bit more insistent than its strength. This is the image we have when we read about Pat's mom. Pat indicates that there were many times when it seemed like her mom wanted to break down, to disintegrate under the strain, but she did not. Somehow, she continued on with the care-giving tasks that had fallen to her to carry.

These tasks were only part of Pat's mom's charge, though. In addition to nursing her own mother through mental illness and unto death, and then caring for an ill sister whose life had imploded, Pat's mom also had a family of her own to nurture. In this sense, Pat speaks loudly about the figure her mom cut for her, not merely in terms of how she bore the incredible strain of caring for a family in crisis. Pat learned some vital lessons from her mom. Specifically, she learned she should dream big and not cede those dreams to a false sense of practicality. She also learned self-reliance and independence. Some of the things she learned, though, seem to speak directly to cultural oppression. She learned that one must work hard for everything one wants, although it is certain that such a lesson is hardly a universal one. She learned that women have an important role in society and that they are not necessarily relegated to the role of housewife. Pat's mom, though, as one who embodies these lessons, is not merely a mighty oak for her family; she is also a healer. In both senses, then, Pat's mom is a hero in the truest sense.

Lindsay's Mom: Grace Personified

"Don't do what I do. Do what I say." Leadership, teaching, mentorship … parenthood and so on: without question the challenge of stewardship of another person's life and actualization is one of the most formidable ones we can assume. Failure in the shape of inconsistency is more than a constant possibility. It is a frequent reality for many of us. But when a parent or teacher manages to live according to her or his own advice, now that is really something special. One might even call it heroic.

Lindsay's mom is just such a person. She taught Lindsay the deep wisdom of generosity through her own example. Lindsay's mom made her living working at a nonprofit organization, a place where she came into contact with people in desperate need so often that she took to stocking her office with snacks and drinks to give away to those in need. Occasionally, she gave money from her own personal funds to help those she served.

And the lessons she lived were learned well. Lindsay tells of a time when she was a teenager and had spied a coat she wanted. She had a coat, but she desired the new one because it was pretty. Her mom's example spoke loudly for her, though. A family without sufficient resources to provide their own daughter a winter coat had come into the office. Instead of keeping the pretty, new coat, she gave it to the family in need, a powerful example of the old adage, "actions speak louder than words."

Lindsay tells about how her mom taught her to be generous, but Lindsay's mom did much more than instruct her. The lesson Lindsay learned was deeper than merely that "generosity is good." She learned that "giving to people is one of the most important aspects of life," that giving is edifying, healing, transforming and uplifting. Lindsay's mom is virtuous in an Aristotelian sense: she not only practices generosity; she cultivates that quality in others. Generosity was part of her internal fabric at the core of who she is.

Mark's Mom: The Great Inspirer

To be a hero, one need not bleed; to love in fullness one need not shatter. A time for bleeding may come, but it is not a necessary condition for heroism. Mark is the first person in his family to go to college. He is where he is, he tells us, because of his mom. No, his mom did not sell her blood or pawn a kidney to get the money to pay his tuition and fees. She lifted him up. She inspired him. She believed in him, perhaps at a time when Mark had difficulty believing in himself.

There is a clear shape to the inspiration Mark's mom provides. Mark is accustomed to hearing wonderful things about his mom from others. She is held in high esteem by others in her community for her wise and giving nature. When a person of capacity, well regarded by others, in turn holds *you* up as good and beautiful, it is difficult not to believe her. Her honoring of Mark was not limited to inspiration. When he would have difficulty with homework, Mark's mom would sit with him and help. She still does, he tells us. Her emotional investment in him, fully apart from helping him with algebra, works to deepen the message: do not just become something (e.g., a jobholder); become someone who does a thing that fulfills and gives him meaning and purpose. What he knows now because of her is that he can do whatever he sets his mind to doing. He can dream big, and he can work toward becoming what he dreams.

Moms and Heroism: A Summary

From ruptured discs to gentle words, from battered knuckles to the softest touch, the heroism of Mom can be a truly extraordinary thing to behold. The gift of mothering, the heroism of the Great Nurturer, is also a gift given by choice, and this choosing makes it all that much more profound, that much more transforming.

Family to the Rescue

As mighty as moms may be, it should not be forgotten that dads, grandparents, siblings, aunts and uncles often rise to the occasion and achieve rather more than mere expectation. We have already met some heroes from students' families: Timmy's brother and Andrew's uncle are just a few examples. There are many more. See for yourself.

Sally's Dad: Superdad

When Sally's dad met Sally's mom, Sally's mom was pregnant with another man's child. Sally tells us that her dad let others think that the child was his so as to protect everyone's dignity. The rest of the siblings followed in quick succession. Too quick, perhaps, for Sally's mom. She took up with another fellow when the youngest of four was still in diapers. Sally's dad was left by himself with four young children to raise. Sally reminds us all that her dad could have chosen to follow suit and abandon the children. Not only did he not abandon them, he and his mother raised the four children in exemplary fashion. Sally speaks about how moms of the other kids in school were envious of the creases Sally's dad starched into his children's school uniforms. Her dad sat every night with the four children and helped them with their homework. In truth, he poured himself into their growth. Theirs were the only homework papers with distinctive lines separating out vocabulary words. On the most intimate level, his children were *his* homework.

He cooked dinner every night and had breakfast ready for them every morning. He showered them with Flintstone's vitamin pills and took them camping and to car shows. He was in the crowd at the children's sporting events. He was their biggest fan.

Sally, a single mom, is finishing school while working and raising her two children. When friends and colleagues ask her how she does it all so handily and with such grace, she tells them that she had the very best teacher. The heroism she idolizes in her dad has become the heroism she, having made it her own, bears into the world.

Agatha's Brother: A Word That Saved a Life

College did not go precisely as planned. Sleeping off a buzz at a friend's house, Agatha was awakened by a stranger forcing himself upon her. Brimming with confidence and optimism until that moment, Agatha became withdrawn, depressed and sullen. In truth she had been broken by the sexual assault, to the point of thinking about ending her own life. Suicide was appealing, only it took more commitment and energy than she could seem to muster.

That summer was hotter than most, and hotter still for Agatha, but her oppressive summer yielded to kinder autumn and school began again. One morning her parents asked her to drive her younger brother to school. Sibilant silence reigned in the car. At some point in the drive, Agatha's brother slayed the silence along with the dragons hiding in it. "Hey, Sis. I love you." She may not have felt worthy of life, but her death would be an unparalleled act of violence against her brother, so she came to realize it was no longer a possibility. Her brother's words of affection and loved became a bridge for her to find her way back.

We do not hear Agatha's story beyond this point. Clearly, she attended a university and worked actively to advance her education. Whether she has wrestled ably the rest of the demons with which she shared an address is unknown. What we do know, though, is that the most formidable monster among the many battering her was felled by a 13-year-old boy who was her brother. His weapon, a single phrase: "I love you."

Michelle's Son: Out of the Mouths of Babes

Sometimes we raise our children, and sometimes they raise us. Michelle was in the army serving overseas when she found out she was pregnant. Being a mom was not in the plan. Her sergeant sent her back stateside to be with family while she made her decision whether or not to carry her pregnancy to term. It was as if a strong timber had been added to her ship mid-voyage. Upon his arrival, Michelle's son changed the center of gravity of her family and gave it a new strength and stability. Not long after his birth, Michelle's grandmother fell ill, but the cohesive force of Michelle's son kept her going and happy.

Michelle's son is in the habit of saying things that stop his family members in their tracks. Michelle was feeling down about something when her son challenged her: "Mommy, you are a big girl. You need to pull yourself together." He offers encouragement when called for, too: "You are the most beautiful mommy in the world!"

His actions mirror his words, though. Michelle's son overheard his grandmother complaining to a family friend about the size of her energy bill. Without a moment's pause he brought her all of the proceeds from his lemonade stand. After the January 2010 earthquake that shattered Haiti, Michelle's son pressed his mom continuously to adopt a Haitian orphan.

James' Stepdad, Orin

The role of stepparent is a vital and demanding one. When he was seven years old, James met his dad, Orin. James did not know his biological father and had no father figure in his life until Orin and James' mom began their relationship. Orin was raised in a rather big, Baptist home. As soon as James' mom and Orin were married, Orin asked James if he wanted to call him "dad," and, without hesitation, James agreed. Orin's many siblings adopted him as well, and right away James was brought into the family fold and was treated as Orin's own son. Orin's love banished any interest James may have had in meeting his biological father.

When James was around ten years old, his mother became heavily involved in substance abuse. She disappeared for months at a time. She wrapped the car Orin had given her around a telephone pole and was in a coma for many weeks. Although Orin had had enough as a spouse, he did not abandon the family. He paid for her drug treatment and counseling, fed and clothed James, and even paid for his college education. James observes rather candidly that Orin took a job that no one else wanted – the job of James' dad. Although he might have felt fully justified to do so, Orin did not set aside the role of dad when he relinquished the role of husband. Instead he honored his commitment to James, and even aspects of his bond to James' mother.

David's Dad

"When I was young, I knew of him but rarely saw him…" Describing his father in this fashion, it might seem difficult to understand at first why David might point to his father as his hero. David seems to understand intuitively, though, that overcoming something can be as heroic as excelling. David's dad has done both, it would seem. David's dad lost his parents in a car accident when he was a boy. His mother was killed in the crash and, as a result, his dad crawled into a bottle in an attempt to cope. David's dad had an older brother, but he was busy raising a family of his own. Care for David fell to his grandparents.

David's dad and his brother inherited a business from their father. Put another way, they helped build the company and, after a protracted struggle, finally wrested it from the inept hands of their father and stepmother. The two brothers were eventually able to sell their business for a handsome sum. It was at this point that David's dad and David were able to reconnect. Not only did David's dad begin to build a relationship with David, he also began to become more engaged in the community. He organized fundraisers for families who had little, and gave of himself as needed. David's girlfriend was also raised in difficult circumstances. His dad gave of himself to her as readily as he now did to all the youth who were in need in their community. David describes his dad's generosity in superlative terms.

It is a tendency among more than a few human beings who have risen to some measure of achievement despite challenging conditions to view with a critical eye others' suffering as a result of unfortunate circumstances. The urge to tell others to "grab-your-own-bootstraps" and make your own conditions better can be rather compelling. This sentiment is encouraged by the view of some forms of capitalism in which we are taught to operate which asserts that anyone can rise to financial security, if only he or she puts in the hard work. Moreover, David's dad's experience might give him some very personal reasons to believe this narrative, to the point of imposing it on others. In short, and for more than a few reasons, someone who comes from hardship and rises above it, like David's dad, might feel justified not giving of themselves to others. It may even seem as if it is a strange kind of compassion, perhaps a "tough love," to withhold assistance. There can be some measure of wisdom in such a reasoning, but far more typically this argument is made merely as an apologia, and only works to justify one's own self-interest and too often, selfishness. Such is not the case with David's dad. He overcame crushing childhood conditions and professional challenges in his young adulthood. After accomplishing financial stability, he might have turned inward and taken care of only himself. Instead, he turned outward and gave of himself freely and selflessly. Heroes excel. Heroes sometimes just manage to rise above. Some heroes do both.

Susan's Cousin

Heroes often inspire us as examples of how we should live our lives. The proximity that family membership provides can give us vantage points into circumstances we might not otherwise appreciate. Susan has just such a vantage point, being cousins with someone with cerebral palsy. Christina, Susan's cousin, has been wheelchair-bound since she was a toddler. Intellectually gifted and formidably capable, because of her condition, Christina needs help using the bathroom and cleaning herself. Instead of being defeated by a twisted sense of indignity that might arise from someone so capable needing such basic assistance, she somehow found the humor in her circumstances.

But humor is not the only concrete sign of her heroism. Christina has earned her college degree, secured a job that utilizes her capacities and is even working to find ways to live on her own, with only minimal assistance.

The extent of the relationship between Susan and Christina is not entirely clear, but they need not be excessively close for Christina's example to be inspiring. Susan tells us she has carried Christina's example with her through her own life challenges. And we have reason to be grateful to Christina, and also to Susan for sharing Christina's story with us; in this way we too benefit from another's proximity to heroism.

Jack's Grandmother

Some of us navigate hard times and, on the far side of difficulty, decide to live life in ways that make things easier for others. Some of us teach wisdom through words but then also honor wisdom in action. It seems that Jack's grandmother did all of these and then some.

Born during the Great Depression, Jack's grandmother knows firsthand the hardship that comes from deprivation. Her young adulthood was not appreciably easier; she was a single parent for three children. She not only managed to feed and clothe them but put them all through college. Jack's grandmother emphasized the value of education, although she herself never had the opportunity to attend college. She was an avid reader, though, and communicated the importance of reading to her children and her grandchildren.

Jack's grandmother is Jack's hero not only because she rose above hardship. She is his hero not simply because she singlehandedly put three children through college. She is not his hero only because she taught him the values of hard work and self-education. She is his hero because she did all of these things. She did not merely say nice things; she lived by principles like self-reliance and learning throughout her entire life and cultivated those same values in others by her lifelong action. Someone just like Jack's grandmother was who Aristotle had in mind as he honed his thinking about virtue.

Mentors and Exemplars

It is a funny thing about hero exemplars – that one might act as a hero without ever realizing one had done so. There can be something of a strange remove between subject and object. It is quite possible, in fact, that the subject may never realize that a hero-relationship has taken place, where both subject and object of heroism, then, exist together.

In sharp contrast, mentors may well be more intimate than parents. After a fashion, mentors are not wildly dissimilar from stepparents. They do not replace caregivers and must be careful not to be seen as supplanting other, perhaps primary, nurturers such as one's parents. They must not seek to replace unless, of course, such replacement is necessary. Mentors give according to need, which means that mentors must always be listening and aware, always aware of the topographies of pain and growth for the ones they try to mentor. Mentoring done with heart and skill is as virtuous a perpetually authored gift of love as one might envision.

Maxwell's Teacher

Maxwell writes, "I think anyone can be an ordinary hero … Many ordinary heroes do not want to be known as such." The hero he names is someone very much like this. He was a middle school science teacher. He made middle school science both memorable and fun, and inspired his students to grow in their understanding of the natural world. A big part of how he managed this was the force of his personality; he was larger than life. He had the capacity to teach to each student in the room like it was just the two of them having a private conversation.

But it was not merely a result of his pedagogical prowess that Maxwell's teacher rose in Maxwell's esteem. Maxwell tells about the time when he was a new student at the school. It was lunchtime on one of his first days in school. He wasn't hungry, so he was just sitting in the lunchroom while other kids ate. Maxwell's teacher saw him sitting alone and not eating. He came over to Maxwell, welcomed him, and said it would be a pleasure to pay for his lunch.

Maxwell had the opportunity to know his middle school science teacher outside the classroom as well. They both attended the church where Maxwell's father was the pastor. In this setting it was clear to Maxwell that his middle school science teacher was as much of a light to others as a fellow churchgoer, as he was as a classroom teacher.

It would be difficult to say whether Maxwell's teacher taught from his faith or chose his faith because of his love of children; either is fully believable. In the final analysis, it doesn't matter. Perhaps, it was both. Maxwell's teacher was a mentor who mentored from his marrow; in great moments and in small he lifted others toward their full potential.

Linda's Teacher

"Tomorrow is a new day and you are ready to face that new day." As exciting as finishing high school and starting college can be, it can also be just as scary. The right words of assurance at the right time can turn the tumblers of our hearts and allow fears to fall away. Linda told us about her high school air force Junior ROTC teacher, a retired air force sergeant, a mentor in ways which he may have understood and in ways that may not have been at all clear to him.

Linda tells about the time when the ROTC team was drilling for a ceremony. She was tasked with carrying the state flag. It was cold, the pole was metal and she had not worn gloves. Despite hating the cold himself, Linda's teacher gave her his gloves to wear during the drill. He taught her values like hard work, dedication and the practice of praising others in public and correcting them in private. He always seemed to have the thing she needed at the moment she needed it, whether it was a timely insight or a pair of gloves.

What Linda's teacher may not have realized is the degree to which his example meant to her. He and his wife have been married for more than four decades and remain as close as ever. She did not have an example of a successful relationship such as that elsewhere in her orbit. Her parents seem to leave brokenness in their wake. Linda's parents are now divorced and had been divorced from others when they got together. They do not get along well at all, and the half-siblings (of which there are several) seem unable to stand each other. Rancor and divisiveness among family members for as long as Linda can recall have taught her that little trust can exist between spouses or among siblings. Her teacher, the retired sergeant, however, has given her reason to believe that trust between spouses can be real and lasting.

It would be difficult to overstate how powerful a simple assurance from a respected elder can be. You can do it. You are ready. It would also be difficult to determine which gift from her retired air force sergeant teacher was more valuable – timely words of assurance or his simple example of lifelong devotion to his beloved?

Alexius' Friend

Jeff probably cannot recall a time when he had both legs. He was born with a leg that could not carry him. Alexius and Jeff were friends in school but were not particularly close. When they were both in grade school, Jeff would get teased incessantly about his disability. At first, the teasing got to Jeff. Soon, though, Jeff began to see the teasing for what it was (specifically, expressions of smallness and pettiness of those who offered the ridicule), and it bothered him less and less. Instead of ingesting the venom or turning his anger outward, Jeff excelled in school. He graduated high school at the top of his class, finished college early and is now working his way to the top of a major international corporation.

It is unclear the degree to which Alexius and Jeff ever spoke about the teasing or about the example Jeff succeeded in demonstrating for his classmates. What is certain, though, is that simply by being true to himself, Jeff became Alexius' hero.

A Certain Samaritan and the Kindness of Strangers

The Officer: Martha's Hero

To describe the relationship between Martha's parents as "tumultuous" would be understating things. Her father taught history in school and her mom was raising the children. Fights were frequent and often as brutal as they were one-sided. It just so happened, though, that Martha's dad's brother was a high-ranking police officer in the state police that served the area. Often Martha's mom would call the police only to have them sent away by Martha's dad. Once he revealed his brother's identity and role, the police would depart.

A particularly brutal fight occurred one night. Before Martha's dad could succeed in ripping the phone out of the wall, Martha's mom managed to call the police yet again. This time, though, the outcome would be different. Officer Jones, a literal mountain of a man, knocked on the door while shouting and shattering were still in full swing. Martha's dad answered the door and tried his old strategy of name-dropping his brother. No luck this. The officer demanded to see the person who called the police. When she came to the door, bruised and bleeding, Martha's dad tried to insist that she was mentally unbalanced and out of control. Again, no luck. Suddenly Martha's dad was no longer the strongest person in the room, and the earth's axis shifted for her. Officer Jones physically removed Martha, her mom and Martha's siblings from the home and took them to a safe place. Although the events occurred nearly half a century ago when she was a young girl, Martha describes with marked clarity the experience of Officer Jones placing himself bodily between Martha and her family and the man who had terrorized them. She remembered looking up at him in awe outside, next to his cruiser. To her, a young, frightened girl, she said he looked like "Superman."

It is difficult to know for certain, but if the context of the assignment (an ethics class in a criminal justice degree program) and the tenor of Martha's description of Officer Jones are indications, it seems fair to assume that Officer Jones' example not only changed her life by bringing her to safety but also inspired her to dedicate herself to justice service. That, if nothing else, is the blessing of the hero.

Orel's Idol

High school athletes often have their idols; Michael Jordan, Mia Hamm, Brett Favre, Serena Williams, Wayne Gretzky, David Beckham, Michael Phelps and the like. Honored for their athletic prowess and sometimes also for their personal attributes, sports idols inspire greatness in others. It is rarer, though, for a high school athlete to be the idol. Orel tells of his idol, James. James was a star of the local high school football team. Orel was a young boy of seven years. After one particularly exciting game where James made several key plays in a victory over a local rival, the team invited fans onto the field to celebrate. It was here where young Orel found himself face to face with his idol. Not only did James take time to speak with Orel at his level, eye to eye; he took him on a tour of the locker room. It was in this fashion that their friendship began.

James had a knack for making everyone around him feel special. He would take time out of his own busy schedule for others. He would come to Orel's school and have lunch with him, and coach him in sports activities. For Orel, James was able to achieve something most adults could not manage – he connected with Orel authentically and selflessly. James saw Orel on Orel's terms and seemed to understand what he was in Orel's eyes: a hero.

Rachel and Sierra

Lisa loved to party. She had a job waiting tables at a local Italian restaurant that brought in enough money to buy food and pot and sometimes even enough to cover rent. Sex, drugs and rock & roll, baby! And that's precisely what happened: a baby. But this story isn't about Lisa. Well, it is more precise to say that it isn't only about Lisa. Sierra was born on a rainy springtime afternoon.

Rachel was raised in a family with a deeply resting moral keel. They went to church because they wanted to. They understood in the deepest part of themselves the message of love and service to others, and more, they realized their values in practice. She was just old enough to work when Rachel landed a job waiting tables at a local Italian restaurant. She made enough money to save for, well, for whatever was next after high school.

Rachel and Lisa became fast friends despite the difference in ages. It would be fair to say, in fact, that although Rachel was almost eight years her junior, she was the big sister in the relationship. When Lisa became pregnant, she was in no way ready for the responsibility of raising a child, and, to be fair, she might still not be up to the challenge. Rachel, though, was a different story altogether. She had moved in with Lisa sometime before Lisa discovered she was pregnant. After Sierra's birth, it was Rachel who did, and continues to do, the lion's share of caring for Sierra.

Lisa and Sierra would identify Rachel as their hero, but this story was told by Rachel, who indicated that Sierra was her hero. Rachel has no formal tie, no promised obligation or bond of blood, to either Lisa or to Sierra. No commitment exists beyond what Rachel chooses to offer. Rachel recognizes her freedom of choice, but in her choice finds no decision at all. Sierra is to Rachel far more than a friend's dependent. She is an inspiration to Rachel, to love and honor her in the most concrete terms.

BOX 5.1 LEADERSHIP NOTES

What's in a name? What's in a title? On a personal level, mother, father, grandparent, brother, sister and so on can be terms of affection and authority. In a more professional or societal context, King, Emperor, President, CEO and Dean are titles aligned with positions of leadership and power. Whether referring to an informal kinship title or formal title of corporate or political status, the well-known fable about the Emperor who wore no clothes comes to mind. It is worth remembering that the emperor in question was still adorned with his royal title even if little else. Titles and designations are more likely to "represent" rather than "embody" a leadership position of authority. Because someone is one's biological mother or father does not automatically infer that they nurture and protect their children. Some parents have to go it alone in the nurturing and caretaking department and sadly enough, some children have to raise themselves, their siblings and, on occasion, even their parents. Likewise, because individuals happen to hold the title of President or CEO does not necessarily mean that their peers and workers respect them or even that they may be little more, than a leader in name only.

One of us used to provide communication and leadership training for agency and administrative managers and executives. An interesting exercise was to have the participants, after considerable thought, write down on a piece of paper what were the four most important things to them in order of priority. After they had completed the task, they were instructed to turn the paper over and list the four things they spent most of their time doing, again, in order priority. They always seemed surprised that what they deemed most important and valuable – typically their spouses, children and spiritual life – were what they spent the least amount of time on. And what did they disproportionately spend most of their time on – their work, social engagements (often work-related) and personal hobbies.

More than once, we have heard colleagues say that work stays in the office and family issues stay at home. Of course, such a sentiment is little more than a bald-faced lie. No doubt, we try to keep work-related stresses from impacting on our families and we do our best not to let family problems detract from our work-related responsibilities. Still, they inevitably do. In addition, much of our adulthood is spent in one way or another trying to make sense of our childhoods. Where we work is in some ways a kind of extended family and, at the least, a neighborhood of sorts. While it doesn't have to be "Mr. Rogers Neighborhood," Mr. Rogers, himself, is, at least in part, a role model worth considering.

Although it has, perhaps, become a bit too trendy as a designation with too many plaques handed out at awards ceremonies, "mentor" is more than a popular catchphrase. As this chapter demonstrates, in both small and profound ways, single parents, teachers, even strangers have stepped into the breach of someone's crisis to provide support and encouragement. That's what a leader does, provide compassionate, even rigorous, care and oversight to someone in need, turning futility into hope and often a positive outcome.

Questions

1   What historical leaders can you think of who were "heroes around us"? One that comes to mind was a wartime President, Franklin Delano Roosevelt, or FDR as he was referred to. When a reporter asked an old farmer who was crying and watching FDR's funeral train pass by if he knew the President, he replied, "No, but he knew me." Can you think of other examples?

2   What does "mentorship" mean to you? Who are some ordinary heroes who have mentored you?

3   Finally, what kind of mentor would you like to be to someone else? Can you think of anyone who could use your encouragement and support?

Reference

Nhat Hanh, T. (1975). *The miracle of mindfulness*. Boston, MA: Beacon.

6

THE HERO WITHIN

At the very core of ethical contemplation is a kind of a presupposed question: What does it mean to live a well-spent life? Over the history of recorded human thought there has been a rich variety of approaches to this question, stemming from different understandings of what it means to "live well." "Wellness" seems to have become a kitschy call for CrossFit among some people today, and spiritual purity in other communities in times past. As a young child, one of us was fed eggs daily until medical wisdom of the time counseled against eating too many eggs because of their cholesterol content. At the time of this writing, eggs are again in vogue, and are even a central part of a popular weight loss protocol.

There is a relatively new philosophical school of thought gaining some support today called postmodernism. Postmodernism rejects the inherent value of grand ideas about truth or beauty, or about humans more generally. Postmodern thinkers like Foucault or Derrida may tell us that we humans have some degree of an inherent nature, perhaps one that desires, even craves certain things, but for a postmodernist, larger ideas about who we are just do not have much currency beyond their capacity to hide acquisitive agendas or affect control over others. A postmodernist would see in our example of the dietary virtue of eggs an analogy for truth: truth, like eggs' perceived value for our bodies, is only about the stories we tell, and about who is behind those stories – who is selling eggs today and what their motives might be. The modernist might retort, saying that all that nonsense forgets the possibility of an examination of the objectively verifiable value of eggs for human biochemical metabolism. We would, of course, point out that our discussion regarding the value of eggs is only an analogy.

Here's the thing, though: the postmodernists have something useful to say, as do those who would advocate for grand ideas, like truth. Ideas can be bent to unintended, even nefarious, purposes, and used to further harmful agendas. It is true that who we as a species can be viewed both in terms of the grand ideas that motivate us, but also as distortions of grand and beautiful ideas, and the agendas that drive them. Ideas of all kinds also come into and out of favor, even ideas about ideas, like Hegel's dialectic, but there are some ideas that remain fixed as to who we are, which remain constant because *they are the very foundation of the existential conversation itself.* And it is to the outline of some of these ideas that rest below which influence the foundation of our being that we turn to in this chapter. The trick, though, as it has been since the beginning of recorded human thought, will be to identify these sub-foundational ideas. They are, it seems, either notoriously tricky to clearly see and understand or, ironically, so frightening in their visage that we simply cannot lay our eyes upon them. Or both.

In our search for these ideas as well as in many of our searches for meaning, we have craved some kind of certitude, some sense of determinability. A settled certainty, a definite knowing, a viewable purpose and direction in the living of our lives are what many of us seem to crave. We hope we can find a rule book or that there is some Best Way to live. Or we may pray that whatever misery we are going through has some purpose. Such yearnings and hopes are as understandable as they can be misleading. About such matters, we have some good news and bad news. First, the bad news: none of us are getting out of this place alive. The good news: we are all in this life together. What is more, we belong to each other in ways that are sometimes hidden from us. We may be our own worst enemy, but we are also each other's best hope. Although we would like for it to be different, experientially speaking, there is no absolute rule book or road map to truth. And perhaps if there were, given our human nature, we might well cherry-pick its directions to fit our biases, thus rendering it useless for its intended purpose. And there is still more good, if challenging, news: there is indeed, something, a Truth, in the deeper realm of our collective foundation, something that is strong enough to bear the weight of us all.

That whatever-it-is often seems both manifestly obvious and inherently just out of reach. It can simultaneously be both frightening and exquisitely beautiful beyond description. It is both object and process, both an idea and a practice. Crucially, it is at least a footprint that moves through human relationships. Such footprints can be seen in the spirit and action of the heroes of these students: generosity, authenticity, compassion and what we might call moral gravity.

Generosity

Have you had the chance to give of yourself heart and soul, to someone? At some point, most of us have. Giving without expectation of return or in response to someone's palpable need can be moments of singular power and beauty. Care must be taken, though; making a display of giving and helping tends to bleach the beauty out of the act. Consider also ethical egoism, the argument that every act, however generous, is selfish. Although such an argument has many supporters, we believe that it fundamentally misses the point. Giving is often a kind of meditation. Self-care is not selfish. It is necessary. It is essential to healing. To distort giving into self-aggrandizement or to dismiss generosity as a special case of selfishness is to in a sense wear intellectual and interpersonal blinders, acting from incompleteness as if it were final wisdom. Similarly, to confuse distorted giving with authentic generosity is to confuse a wraith with a god.

No such confusion is evident among the everyday heroes who graced our students. Let's turn to them now to learn about generosity.

Ellen's Friend, Geoff

Geoff works in a fast-food restaurant. Wages for fast-food workers are, shall we say, modest, and the hours they work can be many and arduous. Such is the circumstance for Geoff: he works long, hard hours for little pay. Geoff does not have much to give, in the way of either treasure or time.

Ellen has known Geoff for many years and has been impressed by many small acts of generosity he has given during this time and always without seeking thanks. There was, in fact, one instance that stood out for Ellen. It came to Geoff's attention that a local elderly man's medical insurance had lapsed, and that this same elderly man required some expensive medications. Geoff used his rent money to pay for the man's medications – for three months – until the man secured insurance. Medical insurance is expensive, though, and securing and keeping insurance are two very different things. Geoff, who was already working a full 40-hour job for a pittance, *took on an additional part-time job specifically to help the elderly man pay for his insurance coverage.*

The old man was at a loss as to how to repay Geoff for his humbling generosity. What was Geoff's reply? "The smile on your face is repayment enough."

Other Instances of Generosity

We have met already several of our students' heroes who exhibited extraordinary generosity. There was Lindsay and her mom: for several decades Lindsay's mom worked for a nonprofit organization that served the low-income community, and Lindsay learned well from her mom's example. If you recall, Lindsay greatly desired a particular coat but ended up giving it to one of her mom's clients. Then there was Helen's mom who, quite literally, broke her own body in an effort to give her children a life that was better than her own. We met Stacey's mom, too. You may recall that she helped run a soup kitchen. All of them gave without thought of receiving anything in return. They gave gracefully, acting from their compassion and integrity, guided by the needs that existed.

Another hero we have yet to meet is Scott's mom. Scott's mother had recently passed away after a year-long battle with cancer. Even during the final stages of her illness, though, she was actively giving of herself for those she felt were in need. Only when she could no longer physically get out of bed did her efforts measurably slow. When she could no longer do for others on her own, she asked her son to help. She directed him to pack her belongings and to deliver them to relatives who needed them.

Authenticity

We have made this point already: heroes do not seek to be heroes. There is no place to submit a resume for the title. They seek to serve rather than be served. Instead, they teach truth through their actions. They bring into being a kind of transformational divinity by the sweat of their brows and the pain in their joints. Indeed, we might say that there is no actual end sought through heroic action, at least not in any local sense. The larger end, of course, is the person served through heroic action; the being healed, the heart mended, the stomach filled. But in terms of the meal prepared, the bill paid or the mentorship provided, whether that act hits the mark is immaterial. It is in the totality of a life of loving service that we witness authenticity. Remember Aristotle's thinking about virtues? It does us little good to wait until someone is gone to conclude she or he has been virtuous, and Aristotle's insight about consistency is not altogether without some merit, as we will see.

Benjamin's Grandfather: The Role Model

Perhaps the clearest mark of authenticity was offered by Benjamin about his grandfather: he said that his grandfather is the kind of person one would hate to disappoint. It would be worse, Benjamin tells us, to disappoint his grandfather than to receive any kind of punishment. To Benjamin, his grandfather was a holy man, in both word and deed. He lived his belief fully; he abided by his beliefs, in terms of not only his faith but also the nobility of work. Benjamin's grandfather preached in church for several decades but was a cattle farmer as well, and as you are aware no doubt, cattle farming is a physically demanding work. Benjamin's grandfather also had fibromyalgia, a condition that involves chronic and oppressive pain, sensitivity to pressure and debilitating fatigue. Benjamin's grandfather ran his farm despite his chronic discomfort, and this alone was reason enough for the grandson to admire him. What is more, Benjamin's grandfather never grew angry or was outwardly hurtful because of his condition. Not only did he not speak harshly, no one had a hard thing to say about or to him. Benjamin tells us that his fondest wish is to be a fraction of the man his grandfather is.

Other Instances of Authenticity

There is a tendency for certain kinds of moments to reveal what is or is not authentic in us. Who we are in moments of great joy – or great sorrow – tends to reveal much about who we are. It becomes increasingly difficult to maintain a charade, say, to fake generosity when confronting, for example, our own impending and inevitable end. In her last days, instead of worrying about her own approaching death in a matter of days, Scott's mom was anxious to give her life's wealth to those whose own lives she felt would be enriched by it. A cynic might retort that she wanted to see her belongings go to good use before she closed her eyes for the last time. The fact that Scott points to this experience as evidence of her heroism speaks instead to her inherently giving nature. These moments were emblematic of her authentically generous nature; she gave because to give was to love. Recall also Kevin's grandfather; he had heart disease and we hear of him after he had lost a leg to diabetes. Confined to a wheelchair and grappling with his own mortality, he would nevertheless have his son wheel him to the front of the church every Sunday and profess his love for his God. Again, a cynic might observe that one's suffering is more reason than ever to implore for God's attention, and it is only a small leap to move from an outright prayer for relief from suffering to praise that seeks to curry God's favor more generally. Professing faith when mired in misery invites comparison to Job, and likely would seek his ultimate outcomes. Instead, though, what is remarkable about both Scott's mom and Kevin's grandfather is that, when facing their own mortality, they *did not change*; they had lived in their truth all along.

Compassion

It might be simple enough to think of compassion as love realized in action (e.g., DeValve & Adkinson, 2008). If we distill much of the scholarly literature on compassion into a single description, we can think of compassion as having three essential parts. First, it is an *act*, which itself comes from at least one (but most likely more than one) *decision*, which is the result of an *idea or belief* (like an ethical theory or religious belief). Such a description is not a definition, of course, as the above could as readily apply to the darker side of human choice such as terrorism or to genocide. An act is aptly described as compassionate when the idea or belief that drives it and the decisions that bring it to fruition are derived from love (e.g., DeValve, 2015). Some thinkers worry themselves about whether compassion "from above," meaning acting lovingly from a place of power or privilege toward those without, is meaningfully different from compassion "with," referring to loving acts that do not originate from a position of privilege. For our purposes, such a distinction does not serve well. One might well take compassion from above to be somewhat less heroic, but it is heroic nonetheless. More to the point, "compassion," from above or not, is an adjective with meaning for the one who uses the term, just like the term "hero." It is not our place to judge the veracity of its use in particular instances but instead only to learn from it.

Howard's Son

When asked to describe his hero, Howard seems almost apologetic about offering what he felt to be a non-traditional answer to the question. Howard's father died when he was a toddler, and he tells us without going into details that his mother would not qualify for any parenting awards.

When he met his son, though, things changed radically and forever for Howard. He became the center of Howard's world. Howard found himself asking big questions about who he was in light of the change brought about by his son. Howard unhesitatingly points to his son as proof in his eyes that there is something larger than any one of us. Indeed, he realized that his earlier major would not sustain him emotionally even if it was more lucrative. Making money became far less important to Howard than choosing a life of public service in a world where his son was.

Howard's choice to commit himself to public service was itself an act of compassion. It was an act that originated from a decision rooted in love. It honored his son, and the rest of us, in a profound way: it is a commitment to a world where his son will live his life. It is, quite literally, loving the world through another. Someone else might have chosen to pursue a more lucrative career, perhaps even at the expense of his own happiness, in order to provide a more certain future for his son. Such an act could also be considered compassionate, but it would have differed from Howard's with regard to the nature of the decision points involved. Both are noble and beautiful in their own right and on their own terms, but Howard's choice reflected a particular understanding of compassion that resonates with us.

Other Instances of Compassion

In terms of compassion, the band "Fountains of Wayne" famously said it best in application to Stacey's mom – that she did indeed have it going on. There is something profound as evidenced by her worries and where her mind turned was, if such a thing were needed, that the role she had assumed recently mattered for reasons other than her own self-gratification. Stacey tells us that in the run-up to her first shift as meal manager, after all the planning and preparation were complete, Stacey's mom worried. She worried about whether there would be enough food, or whether someone would have to go home hungry. She worried about whether it would be a tasty and enjoyable experience for her guests.

Of course, we cannot know her mind in full from the account we have. Such knowledge and insight are not the purpose of this project. Moreover, it is likely that a scientific accounting of the motives driving her worries would be of rather less value than we might think. From an ethical egoist perspective, one might conclude that, whatever her reported worries might be, she worried after a positive experience for her low-income clients, fundamentally so that she would feel good about herself or, perhaps, be well received by the economically challenged community or even by those in charge of the kitchen. Maybe she worried about making a delicious, nutritious and ample meal so that she could compensate for her perceived personal shortcomings. At least one of the authors has had experience working in a similar setting, and has had experience with volunteers who, shall we say, were more than a little impressed by their own kind and capable service to others. Regardless of motive, at the end of each meal, people were fed. More importantly, compassion is a practice (Nhat Hanh, 1975). Like music or cooking or soccer, it is a thing at which we get better the more we do it. Few would seek to invalidate the many honors accumulated by chefs Eric Ripert or Thomas Keller when it became evident that in their youth they were less than skilled in their kitchens. Neil Peart's mastery behind a drumkit is not invalidated because of his having first had to learn how to play. Similarly, we do not condemn an elementary school orchestra for its clear inability to blast out Stravinsky without flaw. Instead, we are invited to see the master in the student and the student in the master. We do not know what was going on within Stacey's mom, but we know that caring for her friends mattered, and for heroism, that may well be enough.

Agatha's brother made a decision. It was an easy one; it was tiny. "Hey, sis. I love you." That tiny decision to say in that moment what many millions of brothers have said to many millions of sisters over the course of human history may well have saved Agatha's life. At the very least, it froze the process of her decaying spirit into a walking wound after her untended rape the previous year. It was not much he offered in size; no elaborate wrapping job was required for his gift. Neither, though, was it small. It was a tiny phrase in a tiny moment, but as a gift it was vast indeed. He reminded her that he was hers. This tiny, massive act arose from a decision. He could tell his sister was bearing something difficult. She was limping, although her knees were just fine. He chose to honor his sense that there was something amiss, even though he did not know what it might be. It is in this moment where we might see at work something of an opposite but closely related phenomenon to Simone Weil's idea of "vesseling," of preparing one's self to listen and tend to the suffering of another. Wounds invite care from another, and it is at least as much in the act of tending, of responding earnestly, as it is in the quality of care given, where healing is in part achieved. Certainly, Agatha's brother offered a powerful gift with his words – he reminded Agatha that he was hers, that as siblings they belonged to each other. At the same time, the magic of the moment was, for her, to be found in the fact that he sensed her pain and acted. He did not have to know the cause or nature of her wound. Its existence alone was what moved him to act and express his love for his sister.

And then there's Rachel. She writes, "I believe that choices … [are] one of the most important processes in molding values and ethics for oneself." Modifying G.K. Chesterton's famous quote, it isn't that compassion has been tried and found to be wanting; compassion has been found to be hard and not tried (Chesterton, 2016). That, though, isn't true for Rachel. Her family members volunteered at local homeless shelters on weekends. They chose to act on their beliefs (for them it was their faith that operated as the source and inspiration of relevant ideas), and so did she. What is truly amazing about Rachel in this regard, though, is that she does not seem to recognize a ceiling concerning her commitment to her beliefs. Whereas her parents seemed to balk at the idea of involving themselves so totally in the care of someone else's child, even though they taught her that their faith was centered on the idea of love, Rachel simply saw her actions as being fully consistent with all she had been taught.

Regarding that ceiling, the limit to which most any idea is subject, Ellen's friend "Selfless Ed" likewise saw none, and his case raises something of a question: is the absence of a limit to how much one gives tied to one's self-interest? Do we give more to causes that, at least for us, matter more? Put another way, do we assess the heroic nature of self-sacrifice when that self-sacrifice is offered for a thing (like one's own family) that matters to us? Is it less heroic to die for a sibling than it is to die for a stranger? Do these links of familiarity or affinity create added expectations or reasonable limits to what we should ask for from others? Remember, of course, that by definition, heroes are people who go beyond even the higher duties called for by ethical formulations like deontology or utilitarianism.

You may recall Simone Weil from an earlier comment that she died for the Republic of France. She didn't die on a battlefield, remember; she expended herself in service just as surely as if she had been killed in close combat. Once called to service, she sacrificed every drop of her life's energy for her country. Now, in terms of causes for which we might give ourselves, we who write this might not be predisposed to give the last full measure of devotion for France or any other country, although neither can it be ruled out categorically under the right circumstances. Then again, neither of the authors of this book is a French citizen, so the expectation of sacrifice in the spirit of Simone Weil is not required of us. France is just fine, and France doesn't know us.

What is truly remarkable about Ed's compassion is that his devotion, certainly offered in high measure, is for someone to whom he is not oath- or blood-bound. There's this guy he knows who comes into Ed's workplace occasionally for a burger and fries – this is the fellow for whom

Ed dips into his own meager resources, for whom he takes on a second job. It is tempting, we think, to seek to link compassion with self-interest. Simone Weil, certainly selfless in the giving of herself, nevertheless gave herself for a cause in which she believed mightily. She was *very* French. In some ways, France was her pathway to immortality. Working to re-establish her proud nation after the cruel usurpation of the Nazis and the Vichy puppet regime was all about her overriding interests and her ultimate concerns. Ed, in contrast, was moved by the suffering almost at the same time as he met the fellow he helped. No introduction was needed or required.

Ed, Howard's son, Agatha's brother, Stacey's mom and Rachel all represent the very best of who we are. It is tempting, we think, to hold their examples before us and conclude that yes, they are heroes and although they may represent the best of us, they may also *be* the best of us. They live compassionately "by virtue of their nature" (this phrase itself seeming to invoke Aristotle's ideas about who we are). Perhaps, they are just better people than we who watch, and perhaps recall moments when we have dodged involvement in the care of someone in need. Perhaps, we can recall looking the other way when a homeless person stretched out a hand and asked, "Please?" It isn't the money, really, is it? It is the emotional energy – the cost that comes with looking need in the eye and caring enough to act– and we just haven't got it right now. Perhaps, Ed is just wealthier in that way than we often are.

Invoking General McAuliffe's terse reply, "Nuts." *Of course* their acts are heroic, but the secret kernel of wisdom we hope to offer through this book is that *you* already have the potential to be a hero. You are a hero to those who love you, and you can be a hero to those who need you. The only difference between Selfless Ed and the rest of us are the choices we make. That's it. There is a "Selfless Ed" in each of us, just as there is a selfish voice. Heroes simply choose to honor and respond to the voice, often the quietest among them, that teaches heroism: generosity, authenticity, compassion.

A Moral Center of Gravity

One takeaway from Aristotle's idea of virtue is that only when someone has lived her or his life entirely, only when loved ones are gathered around one's tomb, cist or mausoleum, can we say whether or not that person led a virtuous life. Only when a life is over can one describe a life as virtuous. Of course, such a perspective is as useless as it is unsatisfying, but we cannot dismiss the kernel of insight out of hand that it offers. There is something to be said, after all, for consistency. It is easy to be virtuous once. It is easy to say or purport to believe nice or good things. It is easier still to be virtuous when doing so obviously benefits the person in question. We are not nearly as impressed by nice or pretty words as we are by deeds that are consistent with higher ideals. Who we are and what we do when things are difficult or, as the cliché goes, when no one is watching, illustrate the nature of our moral center of gravity. Faith may operate as a formative mechanism for this center of gravity, but it is not the only element central to its formation. Further, this center of gravity cannot itself be seen; Its size, shape and power are unknowable as such. Actions are its only testament.

Miriam and Her Sister: Distance Is No Match for Gravity

We have yet to meet Miriam and her sister. Miriam and her sister are just a few years apart in age, but their lives took very different paths. Miriam had a string of bad relationships and moved to the South. Her sister, in contrast, stayed home in New England and began a family. As children they were, as they say, thick as thieves, but during one of Miriam's bad relationships there was a falling out. They met again at the funeral of a grandparent. Things were pleasant enough, but nothing was resolved. Soon, Miriam's involvement with drugs landed her in federal prison. After prison, she and her sister reconnected and worked through their difficulties. Miriam's sister became Miriam's "biggest supporter and the president of [Miriam's] fan club."

We do not know what particular issues, aside from drug involvement, led Miriam to end up in prison. And it would be a mistake to conclude from her having spent time in prison that she lacked a moral center of gravity. What we can say with some certainty, though, is that Miriam was having a rough time in life and that her sister's consistency played a role in Miriam's rediscovery of her own strength and value. It seems clear that although the sisters did not exactly get along while Miriam was coping with her drug involvement and toxic partnerships, the door for reknitting their bond was always open. Even during their period of estrangement, love remained. Sometimes the most loving thing to do with someone we hold dear is to maintain a minimum safe distance until such time reconciliation is possible. We cannot know for sure of course, but it sounds like this is precisely what Miriam's sister sought to do. Make no mistake: although patience may be key, this kind of inaction is not passive. It may seem odd, perhaps, but Miriam's sister waiting for her to be emotionally ready for honest engagement actually put Miriam's needs before her own. It is an active kind of waiting, a vesseling, a preparation. Your bed is made, dinner is in the oven, the coffee is fresh and the hearth is warm. All we lack is you. Whenever you're ready.

Other Examples of a Moral Center of Gravity

Jack's grandmother impressed upon her children the importance of education. No, she was not a product of a selective and privilege-steeped institution of higher education. She was not one who had herself benefited from having an education. She knew that the way for her children to have a life that was qualitatively better than the one she had led was for them to not only attain valuable credentials but for them to invest in their own capacities and, more so, to actualize themselves. As demonstrated by her deeds, she did not seek for herself higher credentials despite her evident intelligence. Instead, she gave of herself so that her children could reach their full potential and be as happy as possible. She worked to support the family and provide them the opportunity to go to school without worrying about food, shelter and safety.

That moral center of gravity is evidenced also when we act authentically, compassionately and generously toward one who cannot reciprocate. You may recall from an earlier chapter that Orel's idol, James, went to great lengths to give Orel the sense of being important because Orel was, indeed, important all on his own. Orel's hero did not take Orel into the football locker room in order to ingratiate Orel to him for the sake of a future payday. Neither did he attend to Orel out of pity. James was Orel's hero because Orel was esteemed in his hero's eyes. James treated Orel as if Orel mattered because Orel did matter. More specifically, Orel mattered to him.

Benjamin's grandfather, like others we have met, also lived by his beliefs. He "paid the bills" of his beliefs when those bills came due. When Benjamin's father abandoned his family, Benjamin's grandfather did not leave them to their fate in Old Testament fashion. He brought them home, most likely at considerable expense.

Conclusion

The heroes that inspire us on a deeper level are not orators. They are not larger-than-life celebrities of one sort or another. They may say noble things and espouse inspirational ideas, but they become heroes when their actions make those inspirational and beautiful ideas meaningful. It is in realizing ideas in action that those ideas become transformative. Heroes have a sense of humility and a moral center of gravity, and they allow that gravity to guide their lives in moments great and small. They don't just espouse compassion; they recognize and honor their inescapable connection with all other sentient beings. For heroes there is no guile, no pretending. Finally, heroes give and rejoice in the giving.

BOX 6.1 LEADERSHIP NOTES

Leadership qualities include the ability to be *authentic* from the inside-out, to learn how and when to speak the truth in an inclusive and instructive (as opposed to destructive) manner.

As mentioned previously, an effective leader also practices generosity, creating a win-win environment whenever possible, an environment that encourages innovation, creativity and cooperation.

Empathy and *compassion* are also essential qualities of leadership. A leader who cares about students, colleagues or employees creates a kind of "we are all in this together" community and work setting. We care about those who care about us and we try harder, go the extra mile, in order to not disappoint them.

These qualities comprise a "moral center of gravity" within a leader. Mark Twain once said, "The most important quality a politician can have is honesty. If he can fake that, he's got it made." In truth, some leaders, like some politicians, attempt to fake authenticity and empathy, especially around election or peer review time. Such efforts quickly wear thin as the difference between what they say as opposed to what they do becomes clear. Authentic leaders who become heroes to others possess a moral center. Their journey into effective and meaningful leadership begins within, within their core being. Over time, they nurture and motivate those around them to become the best of who they are.

Questions

1 Why is it important for an authentic leader, or anyone else for that matter, to develop a spirit of generosity? What are some benefits of embodying such an attitude as opposed to becoming more selfish?
2 What impact do the qualities of compassion and empathy have on others?
3 How does the "hero within" become the "hero without"? Why is cultivating a moral compass within oneself essential to finding the courage to act heroically?

References

Chesterton, G. (2016). *What's wrong with the world*. Project Gutenberg. Accessed March 28, 2020, 8:28pm from https://www.gutenberg.org/files/1717/1717-h/1717-h.htm

DeValve, M. (2015). *A different justice: Love and the future of criminal justice practice in America*. Durham, NC: Carolina Academic Press.

DeValve, M., & Adkinson, C. (2008). Mindfulness, compassion and the police in America: An essay of hope. *Human Architecture: Journal of the Sociology of Self-Knowledge 6*, 3, 99–104.

Nhat Hanh, T. (1975). *The miracle of mindfulness*. Boston, MA: Beacon.

7

HEROIC ACTIONS

It may seem silly to say this, but heroes *do things*. Heroes do something in the world. Even people whose heroism is rooted in Idea (consider perhaps a social or religious figure, like a Jesus, a Gandhi or a Krishnamurti) must at least write their thoughts down for others to read and consider. Most often, though, they also do things. Gandhi, after all, had to *actually* boil seawater in a kettle to defeat the British Empire.

In Chapter 3 we met Viktor Frankl, and we learned through him truly powerful lessons about choice and its capacity to give meaning. We also met Aristotle in Chapter 3, and for him choice was central to the making and meaningfulness of *phronesis* (practical wisdom) and ultimately of *eudaimonia* (human flourishing). Choice, it seems, makes life-giving meaning. Many thinkers have contemplated the nature of choice, of course. Indeed, normative ethics is in many ways an extended conversation about the choices we make, their consequences and how we should understand them. Actions, at least those actions that concern normative ethics, can be contemplated in terms of the choice-making (or lack thereof) behind them. Choice, then, becomes the focus of this chapter on action.

Choice is both deceptively simple and deeply complex, but one thing we can say with certainty about choice for humans (and probably for other sentient beings as well) is that the choices we make create meaning for us, meaning that can be transformative, even lifesaving (for Frankl) and life-giving (for Aristotle).

From the stories shared by Dr. Braswell's students we can see choice at work, doing its meaning-making, life-giving thing. There are many defensible ways of examining heroic choice-making, but it serves us well, we think, to emphasize here two particular aspects of choices made by heroes: perseverance and sacrifice. Heroes persevere despite hardship, and they give of themselves.

This chapter was written during the isolation imposed during the COVID-19 pandemic. Choice, you may recall, was a central topic of conversation. Italy was particularly hard-hit by the pandemic, and the Italian health system was strained to breaking. One of the cracks in the system related to the availability of respirator valves needed for treatment of patients. Under normal circumstances, the valves cost more than $10,000. A group of engineers 3D-printed functional replicas for about $1 each (Peters, 2020). There seems to be a lack of clarity surrounding the details, but these volunteers took on the task of printing these vital valves despite the possibility of a patent-infringement lawsuit. They acted to save lives regardless of potential consequences. They persevered, regardless of potential consequences.

In *stark* contrast, as the scale of the novel coronavirus pandemic was becoming clear, North Carolina senator and Senate Intelligence Committee chair Richard Burr met with big-dollar-donor constituents in February of 2020 and told them that there likely would be significant economic impacts from the pandemic. He then downplayed the threat publicly, echoing the president's message that the pandemic would be akin to a seasonal flu (Mak, 2020). Then Burr sold off somewhere between $600,000 and $1.7 million in stocks just before the market crashed (Faturechi & Willis, 2020) in March. Burr was not the only congressperson to sell off stocks with the threat of market crash looming, but his was the most prominently despicable choice-making given his role as Senate Intelligence Committee chair, his outward messages, his private warning to connected constituents and his own greed-serving choices. The suite of choices Burr made around the novel coronavirus highlights just how important sacrifice, or in Burr's case the unwillingness to sacrifice, is in the making of a hero.

Perseverance

Mark's Mom Again

Mark's Mom we met in Chapter 5. She helped Mark with homework and encouraged him to strive for a career, and to go to college, even though no one else in his family had. Notably, she urged him to value service to others in his personal and professional choice-making. And it would seem as if he had listened; Mark wrote about his mom in the context of an assignment in an ethics in criminal justice university course.

Notably in Mark's treatment of his mother here, he mentions help with homework and general encouragement, but beyond these there are few details on offer. Nevertheless his hand is sure, his choice certain: his mother is his hero. What stands out reading his treatment of his mother is this lack of detail accompanied by the force of his words. Specific events did not leap to his memory; it was the presence of his mother in big moments and small, happy moments and sad, success and failure, sickness and in health. For Mark, his mom is a hero not because she did a particular thing, but because she didn't do something: she did not give up on him. In fairness, she did lots of things, too; she encouraged, invested, supported, believed, inspired, nurtured. She did these things many countless times over the course of Mark's life. Each positive word, each hug, each "Go get 'em," each "attaboy" was a string in the warp and weft of her heroism. She never failed not to fail.

How does her perseverance impact Mark? She led by example, teaching him to lead by example. It would be easy, we think, for someone so beloved to take the wrong message from being so unconditionally nurtured: "I must be better than the rest!" Jokes about races where everyone gets a trophy miss the point that celebrating effort is not about abolishing merit; indeed, it prioritizes it after a fashion. Everyone getting a trophy does not imply that everyone was equally fast. Instead it challenges speed as the sole criteria for assessment. There are times when only speed matters, but it cannot be gainsaid that things other than speed matter when relating to children and physical activity. Seeing success in moments where traditional standards of success are elusive is about understanding need and meeting it on its own terms.

Mark learned the lesson his mom sought to get across: service to others matters deeply, and that it is accomplished through being there; no particular instance wins the day. Consistency matters: every baseball game, every concert, every skinned knee, every A-plus paper, every jilting by a girlfriend or boyfriend. Not failing to be there is heroic.

Susan's Cousin Returns

We also had the pleasure of meeting Susan and her cousin in Chapter 5. Susan's cousin has cerebral palsy and has been confined to a wheelchair since early childhood. Susan's cousin needs help with the most basic of care activities, including cleaning herself after using the bathroom. No, Susan's cousin does not have a choice regarding her condition, but she *does* have a choice about how she lives her life. She could choose to curl up, to give up; she could stay home watching mindless television, waiting for the next meal or bowel movement, simply processing calories. In fact, in this Susan's cousin is no different whatsoever from the rest of us. If we look, we will see that Susan's cousin makes a million choices or more that reaffirm her dignity. In every minute she chooses dignity over despair, capacity over desuetude. She chooses not only not to be defeated by the tasks with which she needs help; she has also refused to be defined by her condition. If you recall, Susan's cousin has not only gone on to college; she has excelled and lives an enviable life by any standard.

We who are not in the circumstance of having a debilitating condition like cerebral palsy make a million choices, too. Our hearts help us: they vote against oblivion between 60 and 80 times a minute, every minute, waking and sleeping. Make no mistake, though: conditions which confront us work only to enhance the reality that each of us chooses to persevere, or not.

Han's Mom

We have not yet met Han or his mother yet, and for that we apologize. Han's mom is an extraordinary example of perseverance. Now, we do not know for certain whether Han's mom is a single parent, but judging from context it seems altogether safe to assume that she is. While raising her two children, urging upon them their own best effort toward actualization, she herself went back to school for an MBA as well as her CPA certification. Of course, once she earned her certifications, it was time to go to work. While keeping her children fed and inspired, she worked hard and ably enough to become a partner in a CPA firm.

All of this would be impressive enough and make her well worthy of being celebrated as a hero. She managed all of this while dealing with a periodically debilitating liver condition. Giving up is tempting when the task is daunting. Giving up is almost too seductive to pass up when that daunting task must be achieved despite hobbling pain. If we asked her, Han's mom might say that she did not see a choice; succeeding was the only option for her children. She would be wrong, though: there is always the choice to give up. Heroes may not see the choice to cave in, but it is always there. It is tempting, we think, to treat this failure to see the option to give in as a personal flaw of the hero. We don't think so. Instead it seems to us that the choice to give up was made very deliberately, but elsewhere, away from the gaze of the hero at least in the moment of looking back. Perhaps the choice was made way back, earlier in life, or perhaps the hero examined possible choices and excluded giving up at the very outset of the situation, but wherever it happened, it was a deliberate choice. Indeed, it would seem as if it would have to be; if giving up were never a choice, it would not be heroism.

Alexius' Hero, Jeff

In Chapter 5 we met Alexius' friend, Jeff. Jeff was born with a leg that required removal. If you recall, he was teased at school by some of the kids. Jeff, though, turned the teasing into something else. The details are unclear, but the teasing became routinized and lost its sting. Many times, perhaps every day at lunch, Jeff chose not to be ground down, not to retaliate. He did choose to make a point, however, and he did so in high fashion. Again, one big choice – not being defined by his circumstances – led to many thousands of small choices, like to reinvest himself *in* himself on a daily basis. Jeff graduated valedictorian of his high school class, went to a good university and, last we heard, he was on his way to the top of the corporate ladder at a major telecommunications corporation.

Jeff's example highlights one more aspect of perseverance related to choice: there are big choices and little choices, and that these are not necessarily very different things. Choosing, say, to do one's calculus homework to the very best of one's ability on an unseasonably warm day in October is, on its face, vastly different from the choice to succeed academically, but it is not different in terms of results. It is the particular, granular choices we make in the smallest moments that give breath and movement to the big choices we make. Wanting to be a pilot, police officer or pastor represents one choice, but that one choice is made up of thousands of tiny choices, each as crucial as the big one. One of the authors chose to begin college at a music school, only to find out once there that the set of choices required of him did not appeal to him as he thought it would; the big choice had to change because of the unwillingness to make the thousands of little choices the big choice required.

Heroes understand the linkage between the big choices and the small choices that make up the big choices. Heroes continue. The big choice acts like a map or guide star, but the little choices equate to putting one foot in front of the other over whatever landscape one must move to arrive.

Hester's Mom: Lifesaver

Yet another mom–hero, one whom we have not yet met, is Hester's mom. Hester's young brother spent a significant portion of his childhood sick. No one seemed able to figure out what was wrong. The rest of the family began to suspect that Hester's mom was concerned over nothing, that his illnesses were just the normal course for some small children. Nevertheless she persisted, bringing the child to a well-regarded medical expert. Finally, it became only too clear that Hester's little brother suffered from a bone infection.

Hester's mom lost her parents when Hester was in grade school. Hester's aunt was only a few years older than Hester was. An orphan at 13, Hester's mom brought her young sister, Hester's aunt, into the home and raised her like her own child.

In fairness, we have seen more than a few moms who have risen to the challenge and have earned the title "hero." Hester's mom most certainly belongs among them, but not only because she has made it a lifelong practice of caring for others. Some years after Hester's mom brought her young sister into her home to raise her, Hester's mom was diagnosed with an incurable, debilitating illness; fatigue and weak limbs became her new normal. What did not change after her diagnosis was her commitment to the wellbeing of her children and sister. Through difficulties with diagnosis for her son, despite the untimely loss of her own parents and despite the reality of a debilitating illness, Hester's mom persevered in her nurturance of others.

Kenny's Mom: Triumph

Yet another new face for us is Kenny's mom. Like others we have met, she has faced adversity and yet remained true to her values. Thich Nhat Hanh (e.g., 1975) likens this capacity to being like the trunk of a mighty tree. Storms may toss the branches about, but the trunk stays still and remains a rocklike support against the tumult. One of us learned recently that several species of trees grow particular root structures – L-shaped roots – that work specifically to stabilize the tree. These structures are harder and more robust than the rest of the trunk. Such a structure seems an apt analogy for Kenny's mom.

Like others here, she made choices to live as she would have her son live. Under normal circumstances, doing so is not necessarily onerous. During Kenny's childhood, his mom's father was diagnosed with Alzheimer's disease and she became the primary caregiver for him. In terms of who she was, the things for which she stood, nothing changed. Not long after she was diagnosed with breast cancer. Many things changed in her life of course, but nothing changed – she continued to live by her beliefs and to teach her son to do the same.

Something *did* change, though; she realized that she wanted to serve more significantly the community that helped her navigate her difficulties, to live her values more completely. She went back to school and earned an advanced degree in emergency management. Now she works as an incident commander while also teaching grade school.

Kenny's mom is yet another example of perseverance. She lived her truth through adversity, teaching her son carefully by her own example. But her own example shows that one can persevere while changing; her own brush with mortality brought to her attention her need to nurture in a more extensive and skillful way those around her. Perseverance does not mean one must remain unchanged or unwilling to be reflective. Kenny's mom represents a shining example of how one can persevere and also change at the same time.

Conclusion

They say that the skies over Shanghai and Beijing are smogless for the first time in a generation. The COVID-19 pandemic might well prove to be one of the most significant events in recent history but not necessarily or only for the illness itself (it seems that Tom Hanks is going to be just fine). Choice-making is the star of the show as we navigate through uncertain waters; choices made, tiny and grand, will be examined and reexamined for their heroism, and for their violence.

The pandemic has clarified more than a few aspects of our culture and our economy. It is from people and their labor that economic value comes. We are a mutual species. Health care is an absolute right (humans under any circumstances owe each other their very best, regardless of the relative level of technology or capacity), *not* a commodity, and it makes no sense that access to health care should be encumbered to, and thus contingent upon, one's employment. There are consequences from choices we make, but it is not sound to justify an inherently violent socioeconomic system around a twisted version of the choice–consequence linkage. If an economic system is shaken to its foundations by a two-week shutdown, then it was a sham from the beginning.

In response to the pandemic, we have seen profound ugliness and we have seen profound beauty. What matters now, though, once the pandemic becomes history, is what we do, what choices we make, from the lessons we have learned. Put simply, the choice is yours.

Sacrifice

The heroic soldier and the heroic mother share something: the willingness to sacrifice, but sacrifice is not necessarily a simple thing. You may recall that Aristotle is some help in this regard; we are unlikely to recognize it as heroic to throw one's self into the lion's den without some perceived benefit. We would balk at the label of "hero" to be affixed to the soldier who throws herself on a hand grenade while all alone. Sacrifice is part of sentient existence, but heroic sacrifice implies a *because*. Heroic sacrifice is done as an affirmation, not as an act of nihilistic self-destruction. Sacrifice is part of sentient existence; sometimes the burnt offerings we give include the hero.

Jeanne's Dad's Sacrifice

We do not know what dreams he had for his future, but when his father's leg was broken by a farm animal, Jeanne's dad quit high school and took over the work of the family farm. The job of carrying a farm is extraordinarily demanding and choosing to take it on so early in life, in effect sealing one's self into a life of labor and relative isolation, seems cruel. Jeanne recounts the family mythos around the moment when Jeanne's dad announced his decision to leave school and to take on the duties of leading the farm.

Perhaps his dream was to take over the farm when he was old enough, and his father's debilitating injury simply hastened what was inevitable. Perhaps so, but at the very least Jeanne's dad sacrificed himself in terms of his own capacity, his own readiness for leading a farm. In addition to being exceptionally demanding physically, agribusiness in the era of sustainability is also intellectually demanding. Even if his dream was to take over the farm, his own ability to move into twenty-first-century farming would be impacted by his early movement into farm leadership; in essence, if farming was always to be where he placed his life's energy, his decision to care for his family under these circumstances meant that he was sacrificing his ability to do maximally well the very thing he chose to do lifelong.

Marvin's Dad

Perhaps the most intriguing response to the question, "Who is your Ordinary Hero" came from Marvin. His father is his hero, and in this he does not hesitate. Marvin's dad took loving care of Marvin, raising and teaching him carefully. What is striking about his answer, though, is that Marvin says his father is his hero despite the many unethical things he has done. We are left without details, but it would seem that Marvin's dad has done things that were unsavory during his life, things of which Marvin is aware. But perhaps we should be more careful with our use of the description "unethical" for the things Marvin's dad has done, things Marvin calls "bad." Marvin's dad has an ethical principle that has acted as a guide for him: family survival.

Just as we are left without any sense of what "bad" things were done, and how truly "bad" they may have been, we are also left without any sense of the circumstances in which Marvin's dad grew up and lived. Perhaps Marvin feels the need to stage something of a defense and justification for his father as hero, but it is a defense he need not make. The inclination to judge Marvin's dad without some sense of his actions or of the reasons for them would be altogether inappropriate. Taking Marvin's defense as invitation is, in some ways, an act of aggression that works counter to purpose, giving breath to the idea of necessity of extreme measures for survival. We might differ, for example, regarding whether breaking the law for the sake of one's loved ones is virtuous; certainly, we can think of circumstances where criminal offending might be the noblest action, just as we can think of instances where it is unnecessary and sickeningly violent. We might also disagree about how to analyze cost and consequences as Bentham and other utilitarians would have us do. In this particular circumstance we have no insight into the nature of the acts, so a Kantian analysis is difficult. If we assert that his "bad" acts, whatever they are, are categorically unethical, then we miss the rather vital point that the reason for them is the perceived protection and well-being of Marvin and his family.

Gilligan and Weil save the day for us; Marvin's dad confronted need – scarcity of resources, perhaps food and shelter uncertainty for his children – and did what he felt had to be done to meet need. We must not miss this point: Marvin's dad might well agree that the things he did were "bad," but he did them for those he loved. We do not know if Marvin's dad faced any consequences for involvement in illegal activity, but the acts themselves represent a very real sacrifice of self for others. Assuming the "bad" acts are illegal acts, and that they are in some way destructive to the wellbeing of others and not *mala solo prohibita*, Marvin's dad will wear the potential consequences of his acts for years in the form of statutes of limitations. Even if he forever escapes legal accountability, he will carry forever the knowledge of having authored harm.

Marvin makes the point that when he was a child he sought to be just like his father. Now, though, he said he hopes to be more. Marvin's dad succeeded in one of the most challenging parenting feats imaginable: he succeeded in teaching the do-as-I-as-don't-do-as-I-do lesson. It was an expensive lesson to teach, and it meant that he himself had to be the burnt offerings, but Marvin learned it while still admiring the teacher.

Extraordinary Sacrifice

Two moms stand out, of course, when we talk about sacrifice. We have met them both already: Stacey's mom and Helen's mom. Stacey's mom gave generously of herself for the sake of strangers; food is love, they say, and Stacey's mom seems to have understood this deeply. Helen's mom gave herself, breaking her own frame so that her children could live richer and less demanding lives. In both cases there seems to be detectable, even from our considerable remove, a sense, believe it or not, of joy. Despite all she has been through, Helen's mom seems to remain with a healthy sense of humor. Stacey's mom seems physically unable to stop singing.

Rabindranath Tagore writes, "I slept and dreamt that life was joy. I awoke and saw that life was service. I acted and behold, service was joy." These words seem almost to have come from the ether; a particular source in which he wrote them is nearly unidentifiable. Indeed, Tagore scholars (e.g., Aruna, 2010) quote this line without citing more details than the author's name. In *Sadhana*, however, Tagore (2020) speaks of oil lamps. An oil lamp contains its light fully within itself, but when called upon to shine it forgets itself, hosting and fueling the light that cuts the darkness. One might give from selfishness, Tagore tells us, but such giving bruises and tears. Giving from selfishness is compelled; the miser pays taxes only begrudgingly because of the gravitational bond between the miser and his money. Love changes the direction of gravity; what was once heavy, once bound to us, is now light. Fulfillment is found not in clinging but in giving.

Conclusion

Heroism presupposed a thing done in the world. Such things inevitably involve a choice; most often they involve many choices. Sometimes those choices spring from us without warning, like Claudette Colvin's choice to stay seated. Some other choices are the result of careful contemplation and take great time and rehearsal, like Rosa Parks' choice to stay seated. In both instances, there were both perseverance and sacrifice. Both women showed up; neither backed down in the face of intimidating authority. As we have seen here and as well in both Colvin's and Parks' choices to stay seated, little choices *are* big choices; big choices are sometimes made of little ones; sometimes the tiniest moment ends up being the most consequential event in someone's life. Perseverance does not mean one should be tone-deaf or stonelike; it means that our eyes remain locked on Polaris, even if we must find a more circuitous route home. Sacrifices made are the last thing from nihilistic. Heroic sacrifice is an affirmation.

It would be a mistake to conclude that giving from and because of love is not sacrifice, not a kind of perseverance. Just because something of the self is given freely does not diminish the sacrificial nature of the act. You may recall Shel Silverstein's book *The Giving Tree*. In it the tree meets the needs of a child as the child grows, never failing to be a nurturing source. When the child is young, the gifts are simple and not demanding. In the end, the child becomes a man and needs shelter. The tree offers herself fully as wood for a home. In no uncertain terms, this fictional tree is, like Helen's mom, a hero: her joy in giving herself cannot diminish at all the nobility of the many gifts: small, large and sometimes total.

BOX 7.1 LEADERSHIP NOTES

We have all heard the admonition that "actions speak louder than words" or, more colloquially, "you can talk the talk, but can you walk the walk?" In the end, that is always the question leaders have to answer to.

As indicated previously, an "heroic action" is something attempted for the right reasons where the outcome is uncertain, a chance taken, sometimes even a longshot. A heroic action by an authentic leader is not an impulsive, poorly thought-out response, although there are occasions where a suddenness of action may be called for. The effective leader is a thoughtful listener, discerning the larger landscape in light of the immediate challenge.

This chapter provides examples of ordinary heroes who "persevered" in the face of sometimes overwhelming difficulties. Even when they could go no further, they went further. And so it goes with a leader as well. If it was easy, perseverance would not be necessary, and anyone could do it. There would be no need for heroic action.

In addition to perseverance, self-sacrifice is also required of a leader. The pseudo-leader is more than willing to sacrifice others, but not him- or herself. We can see ample examples of this kind of pseudo-leadership in all sorts of vocations and professions. Pseudo-leaders are "posers." They may be impeccably dressed for success, be well versed in the latest trends and buzzwords, and be a consummate name dropper, but when it comes to taking heroic action, they don't have the stomach for it. Their leadership mantra, like all charlatans', is "take credit for other persons' successes and assign blame to others for your mistakes."

A genuine leader embraces the moment's challenge, sacrificing her- or himself for the welfare of others and the greater good. Such a leader also perseveres in pursuing a solution to a given problem, no matter how much effort it takes. Heroic action often proves infectious, rallying others to step forward in surprising ways for the good of the community they work and live in.

Questions

1   What are some heroic actions that come to mind during times of social and civil unrest, in wartimes and peace time?
2   Which of the ordinary heroes in this chapter stand out to you? Why?
3   Recall a time that you stepped outside your personal comfort zone and stood up for someone or for a just cause. How did it feel? Were there any mixed emotions? How did your heroic action awaken a sense of courage and sacrifice within you?

References

Aruna, M. (2010). Tagore's philosophy of life – A study of Sadhana. *Rupkatha Journal on Interdisciplinary Studies in Humanities 2*, 4, 504–512.

Faturechi, R., & Willis, D. (2020). Senator dumped up to $1.7 million of stock after reassuring public about coronavirus preparedness. ProPublica, March 19, 2020. Accessed March 22, 2020, 12:08pm from https://www.propublica.org/article/senator-dumped-up-to-1-7-million-of-stock-after-reassuring-public-about-coronavirus-preparedness

Mak, T. (2020). Weeks before virus panic, Intelligence Chairman privately raised alarm, sold stocks. *Morning Edition*, National Public Radio, March 19, 2020. Accessed March 22, 2020, 12:05pm from https://www.npr.org/2020/03/19/818192535/burr-recording-sparks-questions-about-private-comments-on-covid-19

Nhat Hanh, T. (1975). *The miracle of mindfulness*. Boston, MA: Beacon.

Peters, J. (2020). Volunteers produce 3D-printed valves for life-saving coronavirus treatments. The Verge, March 17, 2020. Accessed March 22, 2020, 12:09pm from https://www.theverge.com/2020/3/17/21184308/coronavirus-italy-medical-3d-print-valves-treatments

Tagore, R. (2020). Sadhana: The realisation of life. Sacred Texts. Accessed March 28, 2020, 7:29pm from https://www.sacred-texts.com/hin/tagore/sadh/index.htm

8

CONSEQUENCES AND COURAGE

Heroes succeed … don't they? Against all odds in dire circumstances, they save the day. Is it not the case that heroes earn the "hero" moniker when they achieve the thing they sought to do?

Not exactly. It is intoxicating to view moments like Eisenhower's decision to go forward with the D-Day invasion as a moment of clarity, of certainty. Of course, nothing could be further from the truth. Eisenhower had great trepidation about the success of the invasion, and conditions at that particular moment included choppy seas that led to a tricky embarkation and landing, and cloudy skies meant there might be limited air support. The outcome was far from certain, but the attempt was necessary. Would Eisenhower have been a hero if the D-Day landings had been more costly, or if it had failed altogether?

It is precisely because the consequences of heroic action are uncertain that a heroic action is highly esteemed. If an outcome were certain, it would not be heroism. That also means that heroes may often fail. Some fail until they succeed as we have discussed, but sometimes outcomes are not ever what one anticipates. In this chapter, we will consider the relationship between courage and consequences, and how that relationship may relate to heroism.

Four themes will occupy us in this chapter: faith, meaning, commitment (i.e., example-making) and unintended consequences. First, heroes operate on faith. That does not mean that they abandon the process to the gods; it is not an abdication of care or investment. Second, heroes act for and through a sense of meaning. They create and honor meaning. We must consider meaning, then, for us to understand the relationship between courage and consequences. Because of the meaningfulness of their actions, because of the power of their faith and their commitment to the task that lays before them, heroes become examples for us and for how we could seek to live our lives. Finally, because not everything turns out precisely as intended, we need to consider the impact of unintended consequences concerning how we think of heroes and heroism.

Faith

There is a problem with faith. It is a problem with our understanding of the word. There is both an imprecision and a misdirection in the meaning commonly associated with the faith word. We might, as many do, choose to understand "faith" as a belief in things unseen. We might use "faith" to say to a newly licensed teenage driver, "I have *faith* in you," meaning that the parent believes, in tossing keys to the family car to the young person, that she or he will good decisions while on the road, even though the new driver has yet to demonstrate his or her skill and care behind the wheel with any reliability. We might also use the word to indicate that we possess some measure of confidence in a religious or moral belief. We may not understand why we suffer as we do, but we have *faith* that our suffering has purpose and meaning. One might say, then, that one has *faith* in the grand divine meta-narrative unfolding around and through us. We might choose to contrast faith in this sense with the word *confidence*. Typically, confidence is belief in someone or something that has been proven before but is or shall be used again in the future. One might have *confidence* in one's vehicle, in one's spouse or in one's parent, precisely because in earlier circumstances that thing or person proved its or her mettle.

Such a meaning is not without value in that it provides comfort, sometimes profound comfort, in difficult and taxing times. This meaning, though defensible and more than a little serviceable, is not complete. Faith, Paul Tillich (2001) tells us, is the act of being "ultimately concerned." We might consider what does it mean to be *ultimately concerned*. Perhaps, it means to be wholly invested in one's experiential reality, in the totality of one's being, or even non-being. Ultimate concern, and therefore faith, could mean to be fully invested in one's own ontology, to be all-in with regard to questions of our fundamental existence. To have faith is "… to be infinitely concerned about the infinity to which [each of us] belongs, from which [we are] separated, and for which [we long]" (Tillich, 1967: 14). Tillich is trying to describe faith from a religious perspective, but a big part of his task is to make this idea of faith applicable and useful beyond the confines of any particular doctrine. One need not be Christian, say, or Muslim, or religious at all, to have faith as Tillich means it. Anyone who is invested in the nature of one's own being has faith through one's intent. It is an intentional response and striving not based on an outcome. It is worth noting that what we are exploring here is a kind of "dynamic faith," not blind faith. Dynamic faith takes courage in that it seeks to live out a virtuous intention, even when fear is present and the outcome, hanging in the balance, is unknown. Blind faith arises not from a disciplined sense of commitment and purpose but from the dull and obedient cadence of the herd that most readily responds to fear and emotion. This expansion of meaning of the word "faith" will serve us well as we consider the examples of heroes offered by students.

We might also understand faith as having two distinct parts: it is, first, ultimate concern; second, it is the belief in certain unseen things, things for which evidence is scant or even non-existent. Faith is an investment in and commitment to our lives, right down to the nature of our existence, to bring forth our good intentions into action, even though much remains hidden regarding the outcome.

Cary's Parents

Cary enjoys an embarrassment of riches. He had a difficult time choosing among the many role models he has had in his life. He settled on two – his mother and his father – though he featured his mother in his discussion.

They say that the hardest job in the army is the job of army spouse. Dad taught the importance of duty and of service, but Cary's mom lived these values and more. Mom provided the structure for family life, as Cary's dad was often away soldiering. She was the disciplinarian and also the "fun" parent, which, as anyone will tell you, is a difficult waltz under the best of circumstances. Cary tells us that notably among the many lessons she offered him, his mom taught him the value of faith. Imagine the uncertainty of circumstances in the life of an army spouse: putting aside the fear of receiving the dreaded telegram, the possibility of losing one's soulmate and life partner on some lonely, far-flung battlefield. One never knows how long one will live in one place or where the next duty station will be. Keeping connections with family can be arduous and, often, a one-sided effort. Making long-term plans is a luxury many of us enjoy without thinking. Not so with an army spouse. The capacity to plan a family vacation, assuming resources are sufficient for such a thing, can be a relatively rare commodity, one that can evaporate with little warning.

It is a simple enough statement: "faith gives hope in times of turmoil when the walls around you start to cave in." Cary's simple statement contains wisdom. There is much left unseen and un-seeable for the army spouse, and for the army family. Making friends in school is a thing one does with the knowledge in the back of one's mind that the likelihood is very good, that any given friendship has a hourglass counting down the time until it meets its end. Cary's simple statement speaks clearly to the idea that while much is unknown, faith – remaining attuned to and in touch with one's ultimate concerns – allows one to navigate through relationships despite the lack of lines of sight. Faith is akin to flying a plane using only instrumentation. A skilled pilot does not need to see her or his destination to arrive safely. Heroes seem to have an ability to maintain a focus on ultimate concerns, always keeping an eye on the altimeter and airspeed gauges. More, they seem able to share their sense of direction with others, teaching them to read the dashboard and fly when fog and foreboding roll in.

James' Stepdad

We met James' stepdad in Chapter 5, and his story is remarkable. If you recall, James had not had a male parental figure in his life, living only with his mother until she and James' stepdad met. James' stepdad saw in James the need for a parent – a true parent – someone who would be consistently present in his life, and he more than met that need. James' mother ended up becoming addicted to drugs and would disappear for months, leaving James in the care of a man who was not his biological father. Divorce, it seemed, was a foregone conclusion, but James was to go nowhere. He stayed with his stepdad when his mom left.

In the example of James' stepdad, we see faith in practice in the example of a hero. It is not a faith in something, like faith in a person or even a divine faith. It is faith as Tillich suggests; it is an understanding of what is vital and essential for humans. James' stepdad practiced his faith, his being ultimately concerned with James' wellbeing, by persevering and being true to his promise to care for James, regardless of conditions or consequences.

Now, this last point about the irrelevance of consequences should give us pause. Love is a thing that is offered without a particular purpose in mind aside from the object of love (e.g., De-Valve, 2015). Borrowing inspiration from Shakespeare's *Henry V* (IV, 1), parents do not purpose an end when they provide their love. The purpose of love is the object of love itself and no other. That means, then, that although the consequences of heroism seem important, consequences do not matter in the end where heroic, loving service is the order of the day. James' stepdad seems to have understood this with great clarity.

Miriam's Sister

In Chapter 6 we heard Miriam's somewhat difficult and revealing story about her and her sister. Miriam had fallen on difficult times; a number of toxic relationships, not to mention drug involvement, led to a situation where she found herself in federal prison. It would be understandable, perhaps, for Miriam's sister to separate Miriam from her life; Miriam's sister had children, after all. She would not want her kids to be near someone under the sway of drugs and drug subculture. That was not how Miriam's sister felt, though. Miriam's sister believed in Miriam's ability to recover, even when there seemed no reason to. Miriam's sister believed in her *despite* facts and evidence to the contrary. To believe that Miriam's sister's faith was only about trusting in Miriam's capacity to come back from a rock-bottom existence is to fail to see the real power of faith as a human phenomenon. In a very real sense, Miriam's sister believed in a thing not seen and, in so doing, reaffirmed her sister's own capacity to experience transformation. Miriam's sister could not know what the outcome would be. Whether or not Miriam would succeed had always, to a great extent, been in her own hands, but the stakes were high indeed, with Miriam's life and welfare hanging in the balance. Whatever else, her sister understood this; Miriam's was her mission. Sometimes that mission is best served in a variety of ways and, when the time is ripe for reunion, faith helps that reunion to occur.

Conclusion

Faith is a belief in something hoped for but unseen. And it is also quite a bit more. For the hero, faith is both a gift and a delivery mechanism. It is both belief in the unseen and a kind of confidence, even in some ways a purposeful striving. The confidence is based not so much on evidence, however, as evidence in a human context can deceive as ably as it guides. Having faith does not mean that one knows the outcome. Having faith means the outcome is, in large part, unknown and that the outcome does not matter as much as something bigger and more beautiful that is hoped and strived for.

Meaning

We are beings that inhale oxygen and exhale carbon dioxide. Only slightly less significant for understanding who we are, we are beings that process and trade in meaning. The things we do, say and think are intimately interconnected through meaning. Even acts that are seemingly meaningless – binge-watching videos on YouTube, for example – have meaning. We make meaning in action and in inaction. We co-create meaning and trade in it like an interpersonal and emotional stock exchange. Meaning is both raw material for and an end product of heroic action. This book itself is proof of this: hoping to shape future acts of heroes (you), we have taken past events of heroism as ingredients for forging a clearer and more complete understanding of heroism.

Maxwell's Teacher: A Meaningful Gesture

Maxwell told us about his teacher, and we shared the story with you in Chapter 5. He was a well-loved and able teacher, and it would seem his commitment to education was understandable as a particular iteration of his faith. Maxwell tells us about a particular moment in his relationship with his teacher that stood out, as discussed earlier. Just to refresh our memories, Maxwell was new to the school. It was lunchtime, but he was not hungry. Being new, he had not made many friends, so he was sitting alone without food. His teacher saw him, joined him. He asked Maxwell if he had money for lunch and indicated that he would be happy to buy his lunch for him. We do not know whether Maxwell accepted his teacher's generosity, but Maxwell seems to have understood that the consequences of the gesture – whether Maxwell had the square pizza on offer in the lunchroom – matter not at all. It wasn't in the money or in the attention that mattered. It was the meaning of the act, the gift brimming with authentic generosity where the magic lived. Perhaps, it could also be found in the look of the eyes and kind smile of the teacher.

How We Die…: Kevin's Grandfather and Scott's Mom

How we die is as meaningful, potentially, as how we live. One of the most challenging lessons from the study of criminal justice ethics is the lesson that Job One is not going home. Job One is to serve. Sometimes that means not going home. In death we honor the meaning of our lives, and in death we also craft meaning. Kevin's grandfather understood this well. He lived his faith fully, and in his time of dying he did not change. The same can be said of Scott's mom. Her battle with cancer changed the shape of her ultimate concern – the things that occupied her, but not the nature of her concern. Her overriding concern was to be sure that her belongings went where need existed. To be sure, gifts given from a last will are meaningful, but it is in the thought, the care taken regarding need in the time of one's suffering, that strikes one as truly heroic.

Giving Live Meaning: Michelle's Son and Agatha's Brother

The simplest gesture; the tiniest look; three small words. The epic battles that sometimes rage within us are not viewable by passersby, and sometimes even those who love us dearly may only hear a faint rumble of conflict. Agatha's brother heard the rumble. He knew something was ripping at his sister. His simple words, "I love you," were transformative, and may well have saved Agatha's life. He may never know that, of course, and it does not really matter if he ever does.

It would seem altogether implausible to assert that Michelle's son had any sense to what degree he gave meaning to his mother. His praise of her beauty is not to be taken as a precise treatment of her aesthetic but is quite a bit more impactful than any such assessment would ordinarily be.

In both of these instances the smallest exchange – kind words – made every difference. And in both of these instances, the speaker was in the care, ostensibly, of the hearer. We might expect the older sister or the mother to be the one offering words of nurturance, not the other way around. In this, we are reminded that we are all in each other's care. Through such an insight, we can appreciate how heroes understand and respond to the needs of others.

Examples

We hold heroes up as examples, particularly when the figures they cut are extraordinary, even seemingly unachievable, and so many of the every-day heroes we have met serve as examples to us all. Orel's idol, the star of the high school football team, seems to have had a bearing that belies his tender years. Many such young athletes would be more concerned about the attention of admirers who might provide them with more concrete rewards than simple hero worship. Such maturity would not ordinarily be expected of a young athlete, even though we might hope for it. Orel's idol is heroic, in part, precisely because he bucked convention, because he was genuine and rare in his concern for Orel.

Similarly, "Selfless Ed" stands out as a striking case of commitment and example-making. Ed is far from independently wealthy, nor is he unlimited in either physical capacity or time. Nevertheless, with his meager wages and what's left of his days after work, he makes sure that *a stranger* has the medication he needs. His simple but profound example is not only a humble, inspiring act of generosity but also offers a withering broadside against much of the for-profit ethos of modern medicine in the context of free-market capitalism.

Susan's cousin with cerebral palsy and Alexius' friend who lost his leg at birth both offer extraordinary examples of perseverance, dignity, grace and capacity. Not only did neither of them let their disabilities define them, but they also became shining example to those around them.

Lori, you may recall, had a family of examples. Born to her mother when her mother was only 14, Lori's uncle, grandmother and great-grandparents did a considerable portion of the work raising Lori, bringing her to her full capacity. Her uncle provided early care, taught her to cook and how to use a computer. Her grandmother taught her sewing and hair-braiding, and also that boys were no good. Her great-grandparents gave her a sense of community and brought her into their faith. Lori is who she is because of the examples provided to her by her immediate family.

And let us not forget the imposing figure of Martha's law enforcement officer. He broke her father's violent grip on the family. More than that, of course, his example inspired Martha to make justice her life's work. Andrew's great-uncle also cut an imposing figure of his own. His voice had a force, but his silence even more so. To honor him, Andrew chose to serve his nation as well.

Unexpected Outcomes

Recall the tale of Ajax in Chapter 2? He faced death in battle many times without any guarantee of success or survival. Achilles had all the guarantees: he knew he would succeed handily, and he knew also that he would soon fall on the field of battle. We cannot seem to shake the sense that as a hero, Ajax is more noble.

Heroes do not necessarily have to succeed. What we think will happen when we serve, when we act from love and compassion, is not necessarily what will come to pass. Heroism is not about achieving the end we prefer or seek. Bravely facing one's death does not mean that one can forgo the inevitable. Kevin's grandfather did not hope for reprieve from death by retaining his grace in his final months and days. Kevin's grandfather had recently moved when his health began to decline. With any move, there is often the joy that comes from new possibilities. It was not in a hope to relish his new home that he bore his illnesses with grace but because of the person he was.

Timmy's brother left his family behind in Liberia and moved to the United States with the hope that he would be able to arrange for them to join him once he was settled. As things turned out, he was able to bring them to safety; Timmy tells us about his brother's heroism from the comfort and safety of a university classroom. Timmy's brother succeeded precisely to the limits of his family's fondest hope. Would Timmy's brother have been any less of a hero had an angry and xenophobic president dashed his family's dream?

Rachel adopted her friend's daughter. You might recall Rachel's friend had been busy building up a rich storehouse of bad decisions. The child was the result of a casual liaison. Rachel's friend was wholly unprepared to be a mother. Rachel, you recall, rose to the occasion. Without realizing it, and although she pointed to the child as her hero, she was herself the hero of this story. It is noteworthy that she never says as much, so we are left to see and vicariously experience her heroism. Would we be quick to remove the hero title from Rachel if it turned out that the child lived out a life as loaded with bad choices as Rachel's friend had been? Would we judge her poorly if the child shunned her love and lined up behind her mother to do lines of cocaine? Does the child's life choices obviate the heroism in Rachel's life choices? Rachel did not condition her care when she took on care's duty.

Do you recall also how Lindsay's mom, someone who worked for many years for a nonprofit organization that served the lower-income community, counseled Lindsay to give her coat to a child in need? We can be safe in assuming that the coat helped to keep a child warm against the winter chill. If the family had taken that coat and sold it for cash for drugs, however, would Lindsay's act be any less compassionate and honorable?

Uncertainty, surely a test of mettle in the moment, is unalterably precious. Recently one of us saw an unattributed quote on social media, and it was simply too fitting not to share here: "When everything is uncertain, everything that is important becomes clear."

Conclusion

Another way in which Tillich serves us so admirably is that in his treatment of ultimate concern, he addresses the idea of what he calls preliminary concerns (e.g., Tillich, 1967). Preliminary concerns are smaller concerns, things which seek to stake their claim on us or about which we might think or worry, that are inherently smaller than our own totalities. A chief example Tillich provides is one's nation; patriotism is inherently a preliminary concern, naturally and unalterably subordinate to an individual's sense of being. It is not in one's sacrifice for one's nation but in one's sacrifice for one's friends and family that heroism most purely befits the fallen soldier. The giving is unconditional, given to a particular person, because of the totality of that person.

Heroism is meaningful because it is meaning-*full*. Meaning is inspiration, and meaning is consequential. Heroism is an act of giving, a giving of self to and for another without thought of return or of a particular goal aside from the wellbeing of the recipient. Giving ourselves to each other is an act of faith, of the reaffirming of our individual and collective selves, but it is an act that exists independent from a given outcome. This is not to say that we should not assess acts of heroism, but we cannot understand heroism in its fullness only serving an end. Heroism is extraordinary because it defines as vital the person or people who are directly served by heroic action. In this sense, the least important aspect of heroism is the consequence (meaning the apparent purpose of particular action), because the most important aspect of heroism concerns the person or people served as end in themselves. The prioritization and elevation of another through selfless service is the most vital and most precious meaning of heroism.

BOX 8.1 LEADERSHIP NOTES

Leaders in all professions face difficult challenges in what is often a volatile marketplace. Change is often constant and, sometimes, unpredictable. From competing for market share to managing those persons one supervises, creative and effective decision-making requires that one "think outside the box" – not simply try to replicate what everyone else is doing. Innovation requires a kind of dynamic faith that the chance taken is worth the risk.

The kind of faith that is valuable to leadership is not an abdication of one's values – a kind of whatever works at whatever the cost – but, rather, is found in one's moral and ethical grounding. In order to succeed, one has to be willing to lose on occasion. The pursuit of a course of action in order to meet a particular challenge incorporates a broader and deeper, even more inclusive, commitment and purpose, one where the leader demonstrates both the courage and character to take a well-measured leap of faith. In doing so, a leader sets an example for all who observe and follow her or him.

Questions to Discuss

1 Can you think of an occasion when someone took a chance on you? Maybe it was in a personal or a professional context where someone stood up for you or gave you a chance when no one else would?

2 How do "unexpected outcomes" affect our ability to tap into an inner wellspring of faith and commit to doing the right thing in a difficult situation? What role does doubt play?

3   Courage comes easy when the outcome is already clear and comports with what we prefer. What about when potential consequences seem more dire when the outcome seems uncertain? What kind of courage is required in such situations? What are some examples from the chapter that demonstrate authentic courage? What is the difference between the quiet courage of ordinary heroes and the false courage of those who are brash and boisterous?

References

DeValve, M. (2015). *A different justice: Love and the future of criminal justice practice in America.* Durham, NC: Carolina Academic Press.

Tillich, P. (1967). *Systematic theology.* Chicago, IL: University of Chicago Press.

Tillich, P. (2001). *Dynamics of faith.* New York: HarperCollins.

9

THE HERO'S LEGACY

In thinking about the consequences of heroism and heroic action, we can see clearly that consequences matter not just because consequences are the only things that matter. The aim of action, like winning a conflict or succeeding in business or saving a life, is not what makes heroism *heroism*. What makes an act or commitment heroic is that it honors the person or people being served. What happens next, though? What comes after the hero demonstrates her or his heroism? It is one thing to serve as Polaris for others when skies are clear and cloudless. It is something else to serve when times are tough and challenges difficult, even overwhelming. Heroes also succeed in showing us something about ourselves – we see some of our own potential in them in very particular and concrete ways. Heroes inspire us to be like them, because in some measure, we already are. Finally, just as we are grateful for heroes and their heroism, they, too, are grateful.

In this penultimate chapter, then, as we near the end of our time together, we will consider the legacy heroes leave behind them. Our everyday heroes have provided guidance. They have been more than merely lights for the way ahead; they have also shared the dangers of the pathway. Heroes we have observed have inspired us to be like them. They have become heroes through their own acts of courage, compassion and self-sacrifice. Peace scholars might recognize this phenomenon as an example of what they call contagion (e.g., Barash & Webel, 2018): kind acts by one person can inspire others to be kind in future interactions. "Paying it back" at a drive-through restaurant, paying for the meal for the person in the car behind yours and for the cycle to continue through the line of hungry drivers, is a version of contagion. Finally, heroes embody humility and express gratitude to those who have appreciated them before their rise to heroism. Heroes, too, were once regular folk who looked up to someone and needed help.

Guidance

Linda's ROTC Teacher

There is no polite way to say this: when moms or dads fail us, the injury can often be catastrophic. Linda's parents were not particularly thrilled with her enthusiasm for her high school air force ROTC. Her father did not attend the award ceremony in her junior year. But we should also endeavor to be fair here. From the description Linda provides, it seems evident that her mom and dad had more than a few challenges of their own to deal with. It would seem that they were doing the very best that they could. Linda's dad in particular seems to have been put off by her interests in the ROTC. It turns out, though, that he was an air force veteran himself, and it stands to reason that he might have more than a few reasons of his own to be displeased with her choices. Linda's ROTC teacher did what he could to stand in the gap, though, when Linda's parents could not. He went out of his way to make her feel appreciated and to show her how proud of her he was, how proud she should be of herself. It is painful when parents fail us, but ordinary heroes can often soothe hurt feelings and moments of disappointment.

Her ROTC teacher provided another example of guidance for Linda – in the force and beauty of his marriage. Linda's own family life seems notable for its ragged, discordant, even combative nature. Her ROTC teacher's marriage was a diametric opposite: it was loving and mutually supportive. Linda said that she had concluded that all families were as contentious and mutually confrontational as hers, until she met her ROTC teacher. Someday, Linda may seek to build a family of her own. If she were to choose a partner and maintain a relationship like the one her parents had, she would no doubt end up being miserable. More to the point, she would be blind to the possibility of other realities. Her ROTC teacher's example, not only in terms of the work ethic he taught her, but also in terms of the possibility of a loving and mutually sustaining romantic partnership, measurably increased the probability of a bright future for Linda, one full of joy, nurturance and service.

Lester's Dad

All parents and the rest of us inevitably fail *at* some things. It especially hurts when our parents fail us, but it is also true that when they carry us through a tumultuous experience, it can be truly transcendent. Lester knows just how powerful it can be when a dad is simply present. His hero is his father, and in Lester's writing we can clearly see just exactly why. One of the most daunting challenges in parenting, and one of the most rewarding and transformative acts of heroism, is the ability to be for one's child precisely what that child needs at any given time.

Not too far back, we contemplated Shel Silverstein's book *The Giving Tree*. The tree met the needs of the child that changed as the child grew. The book may well have been inspired by a dad like Lester's. When Lester was a child, his dad taught him the basics of outdoor sports, like how to bait a hook and where to find the bigger small-mouth bass. When Lester was 12, his dad made arrangements with a family friend who owned a restaurant for Lester to bus tables and wash dishes in order for Lester to earn some spending money. When Lester was nearing the end of his high school years, Lester's dad helped him buy his first car. He also encouraged Lester to consider attending college. It was because Lester was in college, of course, that we hear about the heroism of his father.

Alex's Big Brother

For many, September 11, 2001, changed everything. Some things, though, may transcend even such earth-shattering events. Like the relationship Alex had with his big brother. Alex was eight years younger than his brother. Such a difference in age could contribute to something of a divide between them. Such was not the case for Alex and his brother, though. He and his brother were very close. More, Alex's brother was something between a buddy and a father in terms of the role he played in Alex's life. Alex followed his brother around like a puppy dog. If his brother was fishing, fishing was the thing to be doing. If his brother played baseball, Alex could be found somewhere in the vicinity of the local diamond.

On the 11th of September 2001, Alex's brother was in college studying criminal justice. He wanted to eventually join the FBI. Instead, after 9/11, he dropped out of college to join the army. When it was Alex's time to choose, he also chose criminal justice. Although he may have had different aims in pursuing his own life course, one senses in Alex's narrative almost something of an apology that he did not choose to follow his brother into the army or fulfil his brother's dream of serving in the FBI. In fact, though, his brother's love for him still paid off with rich dividends. It is not the goal of a hero to encourage followers to ratify the hero's decisions by making similar ones. Heroes are not demagogues; they do not require others to confirm their heroism by following the same path. Able and compassionate guidance is not about laying footprints for others to fill with their own shoes. Their example, instead, imparts to others the ability to chart their own paths according to their own destinies.

Inspiration

Martha's hero, a law enforcement officer, and Martha herself represent one of the clearest and purest examples of the contagion effect among the student papers we read. His example made such an impact on her that she signed on to lend the balance of her life's productivity to serving the interest of human justice. His simple refusal to be bullied by her abusive father's high-ranking connection ratified her value and the value of her family in ways that would be difficult to explain to someone who had not lived in domestic terror. We are inspired by the laser purity of such an act, even more by the undiluted authenticity of service, rather than by the trappings of vainglory or power. In consistency, in connection and in the joy of service do we find examples that inspire yet more examples. Heroes do not keep the podium for themselves, but, instead, their heroism is a kind of invitation for others to be heroes along with them.

Logan's Mom

Two teens discover love for the first time. Not long after, she misses her monthly cycle. The two teens, both still in high school, will now become parents. Setting aside the rather considerable stigma of being a teen parent in the early 1970s, the difficulties associated with providing for a family without either parent having a high school diploma were considerable.

Logan's mom became pregnant with him when she was 17. She and her boyfriend dropped out of high school, got married and began their lives together. Soon, Logan had siblings – *five* of them. Logan's parents did their level best to provide for their family, with wildly varying success. There were times of plenty, and times when Christmas saw only gifts of Cheerios under the tree. What never changed, though, was his mother's commitment to her family. As a special case of this commitment, Logan points to the educational attainment of his siblings and himself. All of them finished high school and Logan was finishing his undergraduate degree to join the rest of his five siblings who all had earned graduate degrees. Logan's mom, despite not having finished high school, nevertheless emphasized the value of learning.

Logan's choice to focus on the educational attainment of his siblings because of his Mom is striking. He concludes his essay with a thinly veiled scorn for the schoolteachers who judged his mother for getting pregnant so young all those many years ago. He hoped that they could see in the successes of her children just how wrong they had been to hold his mother in contempt, holding her as unworthy of their energies and pressuring her to forgo her dreams. Logan's mom could have chosen to be embittered because of her callous teachers. Perhaps, she was to some extent. Whatever her feelings for her teachers were, with an effort nothing short of heroic, she put her children's interests before her own and, in doing so, inspired her children to greatness.

Han's Mom and Benjamin's Grandfather

We have seen already that heroism is more about how a thing is done, and for whom, than it is about what particular goals are achieved. Two striking examples of inspiring heroes met earlier, Han's mom and Benjamin's grandfather, both worked hard to procure demanding jobs and then worked through pain to succeed at those jobs. Han's mom carried the family while going to school. Once done with school, she strove to earn her CPA certification. Then she earned a partnership in an accounting firm. Through it all, she battled a liver condition that sapped her energy. Nevertheless, she worked 100-hour weeks during tax time to help keep the firm rolling and to support her family.

Anyone who knows will tell you that carpentry is a demanding trade, and not everyone who endeavors to craft with wood is deserving of the title "carpenter." Benjamin's grandfather, a carpenter in the most hallowed sense, was also a preacher. His fibromyalgia not only did not hinder his craft, but neither did it blunt his faith. For both Han and Benjamin, their respective heroes inspired them by simply continuing – persevering, by not caving in the face of adversity. They hurt, they struggled, but they never conceded defeat.

Kelly's Dad and James' Stepdad

"I know that he is a man of his word," Kelly intones, "and I myself strive to be the same." Two men, one a father and the other a stepfather, modeled a heroism more profoundly than Homer could have done with the might of his poetry. Two men who understand that compassion is true strength and that tenderness is highest wisdom chose to insist on nurturance when for much of their lives, the standard for maleness was ruggedness, a benumbed churlishness and physical strength. These two men demonstrated heroism and, very likely, created future heroes (their children, for example) by the fiercely loving figures they cut.

Gratitude

Through inspiration and gratitude, Benjamin's grandfather often emphasized the trope about living one's "dash." He sought to make clear to his grandson that how he treated others during his time on earth was the chief measure of someone's life. In particular, though, Benjamin's grandfather emphasized two things in the living one's "dash:" gratitude and love. It is striking when someone who labors through a demanding job despite an incurable and grievously painful condition, nevertheless, offers gratitude. Benjamin's grandfather is just such an example. He does not rage at God, although some may feel he has ample reason to. Instead, he enthusiastically celebrates his faith.

He is far from alone in his expression of gratitude. Kevin's grandfather also expressed his gratitude loudly enough for us to hear him from here. Maxwell's teacher evidenced his gratitude, perceivable even at considerable remove from us. It is gratitude for the chance to stand beside young people as they grow into themselves and begin to know their own strength. Miriam's sister, a hero to Miriam, had much to be grateful for. After all, she had regained a sister.

Conclusion

Not a few psychologists are fond of saying, "hurting people hurt other people": because of their pain, damaged people cause injury to others, and to themselves. Just as surely, though, we can also say, "heroes make others, heroes." Heroism inspires heroic action. This chapter has been about what happens after heroism occurs, but it would be just as aptly framed as an examination of what happens *before* heroism happens. The only thing is that we do not yet know what kinds of heroic actions these students – or you – will bring into the world.

The identification of someone as a hero tends to set that person apart, above. This separating, though, is nuanced: if the hero seeks the separation, it ceases to be heroism. Heroism is a separation that invites and reaffirms a more pervasive unity and mutuality. Ordinary heroes are in the end extraordinary human beings who encourage us to become more than we thought we could be.

BOX 9.1 LEADERSHIP NOTES

What constitutes the legacy of a heroic leader who is also ethical?

"Guidance" is an overarching relationship umbrella that can be both subtle and nuanced, and, on occasion, direct and to the point. The guidance such a leader provides is more about inclusively getting the job done than about who gets the credit. Inclusiveness translates into including others in both task and reward, while exclusiveness can become a kind of elitist self-branding and promotion, one that focuses more on excluding than including.

"Inspiration" in-spires—breathes life and energy into—cooperation where everyone competes with themselves to do their best, to be their best and most effective selves. Whether the outcome of a task that is laid before them results in a win, lose or draw outcome, the collective community can remain intact, reinvigorating itself and following the example their leader has set for them. While such a leader may be captain of the ship, there is never any doubt that he or she is in the boat with them, doing whatever needs to be done.

The end result of such a leader's legacy is one of "mutual gratitude." We tend to remember moments in relationships more than pay raises. The moment our supervision thanked us for a job well done, the private moment she or he shared a vulnerability that engendered the building up of trust and the unexpected act of kindness and generosity all empower feelings of gratitude on both the giver and the receiver.

Questions

1   We tend to remember teachers more than a given grade. What teacher or teachers stood out to you in motivating you to do your best? Did they exhort you to excel academically, or were they more adept in listening and discernment?

2   Inspiration can come from a single act as in Martha's law enforcement hero or in response to the lifestyle of someone who encourages you, as in the case of Linda's ROTC teacher. You could even consider someone you know who is going through a difficult time who you might like to encourage and inspire.

3   Why and how is inclusiveness an important characteristic of someone who provides guidance for others? Identify several examples of relationships in this chapter where helpful guidance was offered and received.

Reference

Barash, D., & Webel, C. (2018). *Peace and conflict studies* (4th ed.). Thousand Oaks, CA: Sage.

10
PORTRAIT OF A HERO

What, after all of this, did we learn about heroes and heroism? In the very first pages of this book we wondered whether there was more to heroism than what Superman might be able to show us. We wondered what it means for people living today when someone is described as a hero, or when an act is called heroic. The simple class assignment that forms the keel and frame of this work asked each student to indicate her or his "ordinary" or "everyday" hero. What became immediately clear, of course, is that the heroes we met through their stories were *anything* but ordinary.

The extraordinary tales of everyday heroes and heroism are all very well, but what can they tell us about how we should live our lives, and what can we discern about how justice might more ably be done? This final chapter will seek to derive insights into the nature of heroism from all that has come before, and to apply those lessons to the wider enterprise of affecting justice.

Lessons Learned

In this section, we will contemplate some key lessons and bring together the sections of the book: historic heroes, ethical theories, organizational theories and the stories of students' ordinary heroes in order to discern a general shape of heroism as we might understand it today, particularly with regard to serving the needs of justice. We will also answer the questions, either posed or implicit, from the first chapters: Are heroes of a moment or do they make a moment? Is heroism a thing about which we must agree? What is the role of ethical schemas in the making of a hero? What is the defining essence of heroism and where can we see it?

Needing Heroes: Weakness or Wisdom?

Bertolt Brecht implies for us that a nation that needs heroes, that counts on an external force to save it, is unfortunate. This sentiment is instructive, but it requires something of a corrective. If we remove the words "unfortunate" or "unhappy" and replace them with more complete and precise terms such as "suffering," the nation that needs heroes is, well, everyone. And Brecht may have a point in that it may indeed be unfortunate if a nation is looking for a single superhero to save it, but the need for a collective of ordinary heroes seems apparent and essential to restore a nation to health.

Suffering is endemic to sentient existence. Suffering, or *dukkha* in Pali, is the dis-ease that comes from involvement, from attachment to things, including ourselves. It is hardly a weakness to suffer; we suffer because we love our children, our beloveds, our parents, our friends, our students. On the contrary, suffering is natural. Buddhists are committed to the minimization of suffering, but not its elimination. Suffering is a teacher, too; it is from suffering that we grow. Suffering is as endemic to our mortal condition, but so is thriving. Joy and sorry, victory and defeat, unexpected success and unexpected failure, beginnings and endings are each in their own turn two sides of the same coin.

A turn from a focus on unhappiness to a focus on suffering points directly at the centrality of need as engine for heroic action. The authentic hero perceives and understands the needs of another, and that need drives the hero to action in service. It is not unhappiness that should concern the hero. A hero's basic job description is aiding in the transformation of suffering into insight, wisdom and wholeness.

Ethical Principles: Battles Won and Lost

In something of a twist on history, it is not without reason that we might assert that it was Lee, and not Lincoln, who was the purer hero. Lee lost on the field of battle, but his defeat did not compel him to reorganize his ethical priorities. He chose sides and accepted the consequences. It may well be that Lee detested slavery as much or even more than Lincoln, although we could never know for certain. Lincoln paid homage to his universalist sympathies informed by his faith. Only once his superordinate particularist value was, at least for a time, lost. Unable to shore up a union, states tumbling from his grasp, Lincoln seems to have paid homage to what was for him, a subordinate principle: the humanity of nonwhites.

Older ideas do not always provide the energy needed to confront new challenges. As we grow as individuals, so do we grow collectively as a species. Some old ideas weather well and remain sturdy firmament, but others crumble to dust in the crucible of the moment. Agatha's secure world changed in a moment and without notice. Things on which she relied no longer had shoulder on which to bear her. Things, of course, except her kid brother's love.

If we narrow our focus just a little, it becomes clear that Kant's principle of universalism is actually consequentialist after a fashion (see, e.g., Cummiskey, 1990). Kantian universalism invites us to think about *what would happen if* action translated itself into universal law. He invites us to consider what is permissible based on the *consequences* of an action made universal. Two seemingly diametrically opposite ideas – consequentialism and nonconsequentialism – are not nearly as oppositional as we might first think. We crave a firm toehold against the surf's undertow, but sometimes what we think is firm reef or rock reveals itself as shifting sand at the very moment when we need solidity most. It would seem, then, that the substantive nature of the ethical schema matters greatly.

To us, Achilles, the mighty hero of the Trojan War, ends up looking more like a spoiled bully than a hero. He is driven by vainglory and selfish, prideful anger, not the wellbeing of his comrades or the nobility of their common cause. Similarly, like an advanced degree bought from a website, Galahad's divinity is a divinity in name only. Arthur's dirty fingernails are far more divine, transformative, inspired and inspiring than Galahad's sterile hands. Galileo's heroic stand seems to have been neither that heroic nor that firm of a stand, and Alonzo Quixano forsook poor Don Quixote when it mattered most.

But almost without exception, practically every one of these students' ordinary heroes remained true to a particular ethical schema. Yes, they taught by example, powerful lessons: the lesson of perseverance despite challenge, the nobility of meaningful sacrifice, the grace of unconditioned and unconditional kindness. Linda's ROTC teacher demonstrated the value of hard work, of praising in public and reprimanding in private. Cary's mom lived the lesson of perseverance in a way only an army spouse could. Jeanne's dad demonstrated the power of self-less service, sacrificing himself for the wellbeing of the family. More than any of this, though, these heroes *taught*: by both message and example, they invested in the person who tells us their hero's story. They taught. They served. And as Greenleaf (and Tagore, of course) would remind us, service is leadership and service is joy. The everyday heroes of these students seem to have grasped something about ethics that Lincoln, Lee, Galahad, Galileo and Quixote all failed to grasp: the highest – and hardest – ethic of heroic service is love. We can see this highest ethic at work in the unconditioned nurturance of Orel's young idol, Lester's dad, Sally's dad, James' stepdad, Pat's mom and Marvin's dad. We can see it in the bulged discs in Helen's mom's back, and we can see it in the humbling generosity of "Selfless Ed." We might even be tempted to say that the highest ethic is one that rejects ethical systems as such, puts down the book or the yardstick, and simply encounters a hurting or growing heart, just as Gilligan and Weil would encourage us to do. The greatest and mightiest ethic, then, might be no formal ethic at all.

Identity and Leadership

States-people, moms, generals, teachers, soldiers, students, stepdads, law enforcement officers, kid brothers: at the risk of sounding a little like Yogi Berra, it does not matter who you are; who you are is vital for understanding heroism. Anyone can be a hero; there is no requirement that a hero be in a position of responsibility or authority. Such positions, however, do tend to invite heroic leadership. They may invite it, but they cannot compel it. Similarly, heroes come from all walks of life (e.g., cultures, faiths, identities, neuro-diversities) and all strata within organizations.

Identity mattered for both Lincoln and Lee but in a catastrophically cruel way. In something of a similar fashion, trait theories of leadership privilege certain attributes at the expense of others, not infrequently drawing arbitrary lines and leaving some forever on the margins. Heroes come from all points on the human compass, however, and traits, even traits linked ostensibly to capacities, offer rather less horsepower for doing the work of organizations, like police or sheriff's departments or state prisons.

For example, regarding the example of Galileo, we heard Feyerabend's insights regarding the nature of expertise. The Galilean–Ecclesiastical conflict was more about how expertise should operate in the human sphere. It would seem that today, we do better for ourselves when we understand both approaches – both the purity of some kinds of knowing and the necessity of the contextualization of other kinds of knowing. No one is arguing that the scientific discovery of gravitational waves must be lensed through Rabbinical wisdom or Pure Land Buddhist doctrine, but it would just as impertinent to assert that social scientific findings should be held without determining their relevance for improving the lived experiences of humans. There are different kinds of knowing, different kinds of expertise. And if there are different kinds and ways of knowing, then it stands to reason that there are a variety of ways of doing any particular thing that might interest us (say, for example, social and criminal justice service). We seem to understand this reality far better than Galileo and his contemporaries did, even if we grant the assumption that they were tuned in to this aspect of their circumstances, but it cannot be said that we have learned this lesson fully.

For example, the inspired courage of Claudette Colvin should have been more than sufficient to dramatize the violence being visited upon African-Americans in the south. Sadly, for white middle-class northerners of the time to be able to process the brilliant beauty of her act, the dignity (and perhaps complexion) of a Rosa Parks was necessary to make it more palatable for white audiences. Colvin's inspired and unmediated knowing and Parks' strategized and contextualized knowing were both necessary to be effective in inspiring change.

In the section in Chapter 2 that focused on Henry V, we wondered whether it is meaningful to call someone a hero whose personage is so deeply divisive as was Henry, or perhaps Joan of Arc? Would the French of the time have been as likely as their English contemporaries to call Henry V a hero? And what would the English say of Joan of Arc? Not everyone will agree on the bestowal of the title "hero" on every example we might produce, but it seems as if at least some measure of agreement matters here. Bestowing the hero title on someone so divisive as Henry V is more likely to be a rhetorical act than an honest assessment of her or his exceptional nature in a broader sense. The English might thrill to call Henry V a hero, but we are under no compulsion to agree. Both authors recall a time, for example, when Christopher Columbus was universally hailed as a navigational explorer and hero.

It does not matter who you are – your identity categories cannot constrain your heroism. At the same time, your identity, your roles matter deeply. Family members, like Lori's family, Gary's mom, Lindsay's mom and David's dad, carry a particular burden, but often it is a yoke they assume with joy. Public servants, like Martha's law enforcement officer, bear a weighty yoke of duty as well, but it is one for which they are trained, equipped and supported. Strangers carry a responsibility, too, but it is a more ethereal burden. It is a burden with its taproot in belief, compassion and in mutuality.

And lest we forget, how you as "hero" is yours and yours only. Your capacity to "hero" is strongest only when you "hero" authentically from who you are. The corollary to this insight is that heroism begins within; heroes know themselves, and from the bedrock of their own sense of self, can they push into the surf and drag another to safety. In the end, you are your own firmament, but it is a firmament because you belong to the rest of sentience, the one among many.

Meaning

Viktor Frankl survived an experience that would (and did) kill the considerable majority of the people who experienced it. He survived, if you recall, because of meaning. He had something that he felt in the deepest part of himself that had to get done. It could not wait for someone else to do it. He *needed* to do it. He carried that task with him; it was perhaps, a shield of sorts, but crucially, it was *not* sword. He did not emblazon his task's crest on a flag and plant it on a barricade. It was a justification for survival, but not a justification to destroy another, no matter how reprehensible the others' actions or how wretched their heart. His project, the thing he had to do, was to write. He had to tell his story which in an intimate way, was also humanity's story of meaning and survival (*Man's Search for Meaning*).

It seems clear that although it was the task that gave him meaning, and that meaning was for him a lifeboat, behind and below the power of the meaning of the task for him, it was not so much the task that mattered, but him. Whether he recognized it fully or not, *he*, his life, was the meaning. Music is just one bandwidth of meaning. Music does not live inside the violin, though the violin is the foil for its creation. The music lives within the musician and works in the space between the musician and the audience. The lifesaving meaning to which Frankl points, like Janus and like theory done well, points two ways at once. Frankl's intellectual projects were intended to weave a transformative narrative for others, but at the same time, they point back to him and highlight that perhaps, the more authentic meaning of his project, the real floatation device, was he himself. But just as meaning is shield and not sword, the meaning resides not only in the ideas or the works that contain them but also in the person himself. Michelle's son gave meaning to her life; he is a hero without ever having intended to be such a thing, but quite clearly, *he* is the meaning which he gave.

It can be seen, then, that heroes are both of a moment and also make moments. It is a distinction without a difference; heroes leverage moments and heroes craft moments, and of course, it is extraordinary moments and circumstances that call forth to them and draw them in. What we should keep close in mind, though, is that it is the meaning of the moment that matters most of all. More than the meaning contained in powerful ideas are the sentient beings who offer and who serve and sacrifice themselves in the heroic moment.

A Kingdom of Ends

The end of heroic action is precisely what makes heroism heroic, even if the particulars matter little, or at all. Arthur's mythical dirty fingernails, and those very real ones of Helen's mom, are where we find heroism in its most genuine form. But it is not in the dirt or in the work they represent where heroism can be found.

The particular tasks we do when we serve are the least important part of heroism; far more crucial is that the act of service itself coronates the person or people served as ends themselves. It is as if Arthur crowns his own subjects with his own crown. On one side of Arthur's blade Excalibur was the engraving, "Take me up." On the other side was engraved, "Cast me away." The authentic hero, especially the ordinary one, like the noble king, is a servant leader.

By what means can such a leadership be realized? A central skill for servant leadership is listening, and we have seen perhaps, the most refined version of skilled listening in Simone Weil's idea of "vesseling." Vesseling is the process whereby a future hero prepares her- or himself to receive, to listen to the needs of another. The hero is not fully transparent; however; the hero embodies heroism by serving from two sources of inspiration: first, the hero acts from what was learned through vesseling; second, the hero has his or her own capacities to bring to bear on the task of service. Heroism seems to arise from the place where vesseling and innate capacity overlap.

The Problem and Power of Choice

Heroes make heroic choices, but it seems that should go without saying. How, though, are we to understand the nature of the choices that lie behind and within heroism?

The heroic choice is both compelled by need and also fully voluntary at the very same moment. Perceived need is only an invitation to action. It is in the active choice to serve, the choice to give of one's self for the sake of others, that heroism truly has meaning.

Don Quixote's double vision was not a madness, although it appeared to be so from the outside. He was not powerless to the romantic novel tripe stacked high in his office, and the purging fire offered no respite. The other world he saw, the noble world, was a very deliberate choice. The choice can be seen at the end where, on his deathbed, Quixano does more to Don Quixote than any enemy defeat could ever do. He denies him. Quixano chooses to return to the distorted truth of reality. Pat's mom chose repeatedly to nurture those around her, to confront the considerable and, at times, overwhelming need she saw on all sides: her mother, all the way through to her moments of agony; her sister, fighting cancer and losing her husband to violence; her children during their formative years. Pat's mom did not have to do all that she did, and yet she would argue (as evidenced by her actions as we receive them) that the choice to care for her family, in sickness and in health, was made long ago.

Composite Sketch of an Ordinary Hero

First things first: a hero must prepare him- or herself. Likely it will look different for each hero, but some form of preparation, even a kind of transformation, is antecedent to heroism. Arthur and Don Quixote, like new parents, had transformative moments of great significance and heightened awareness. Almost certainly, Sally's dad remembers the moment of Sally's birth in vivid detail. Logan's mom has six children, but without doubt she can recall the transformative and unique circumstances of at least part of each child's entry into the world. Preparation takes many forms, but through becoming prepared, we can become mighty oak trunks like Pat's mom, as well as supple, agile and fluid like Kelly's and Lester's dads, addressing needs as they arise. Weil reminds us of the importance, and of the power, of vesseling – being present and listening in order to serve with fullness of insight and precision. Preparation need not be a sudden, lightening-strike moment; quiet contemplation in the solitude of one's own heart and inner being often occurs without any external, apparent manifestation.

Preparation looks like many things: it can be the crucible of childbirth or the active stillness of meditation. It can be the deliberation at a Maritzburg train station (e.g., DeValve, 2015) or the inspired in-the-moment decision to offer a no that ratifies a more transcendent yes, like Claudette Colvin made.

Second, heroes perceive need. Having prepared, having listened, heroes see and understand to the greatest extent possible, the nature of need that confronts them. Need-perception is the first of the three-part process of heroic action. Third, heroes understand mutuality with another. The perception and understanding of need represent the first of three parts of heroic action. Perception and understanding alone do not necessarily compel heroic acting; it is from the realization of our mutuality. Fourth, heroes act. They make choices, but these choices are powered both by their own preparation and by what they have come to understand about themselves, about the need that is at hand, and about mutuality.

Finally, heroism is contagious. Beneficiaries of heroism today become tomorrow's heroes. Tagore's metaphor of the lamp serves to illustrate how the components of the composite sketch of a hero work together. Preparation is the filling of the lamp with oil. The darkness that surrounds those in the room represent the need as perceived; that all in the room confront the same darkness is the realization of mutuality. The match stands in for the decision, the choice to act according to need and capacity, and, quite simply, the light from the lamp that is lit, is heroism.

Relevance for Criminal Justice Practice in America

If we were to take a straw poll among criminologists, professional assertions on the question would vary widely: "Is the American criminal justice system broken?" Some might say so, that it is terribly broken, and point as evidence to the many kinds of harm done wantonly in the name of justice or by those charged with the trust of public service. Others would assert that although problems exist, the justice system works tolerably, sometimes even admirably, well. Yet another group of criminologists will agree with the latter that the system works as intended, but their agreement is a critique more scathing than that offered by the first group. This third group of criminologists would say that the harm done, for example, to Black lives and other minority communities, is intentional, and that the criminal justice system is too often a tool for oppression. That many justice professionals have no intention to oppress, and work their entire careers in good faith does not necessarily put the lie to the idea that justice practice exists as an apparatus for oppression. Indeed, these criminologists might contend that the system works as it does precisely to provide a degree of diffusion of responsibility for the racethnic and class oppression it is designed to perpetuate.

There might also be a fourth group of criminologists, and it is this group into which the authors tend to fall, a group frustrated by catastrophic failures of justice like the killing of scores of humans like George Floyd, Breonna Taylor, Amadu Diallo, Tamir Rice and Michael Brown, or the breath-stopping graft of the Baltimore Gun Trace Task Force. These criminologists understand that there are systematic biases in justice institutions that consistently protect some and condemn others, that merges individual catastrophe and systematic violence into wider and flaw-riven fabric: *mediocracy*. Mediocracy is a single-word critique; it is mediocre government led by the mediocre, where the mediocre persons of middling quality or potentially biased policy is commended. It embodies the failings of a justice system in which individuals continue to do human damage. In such an environment, institutions cannot ever quite seem to address the apparent needs of social and criminal justice and commit themselves to make the hard choices and do the necessary work of social and institutional change. Instead, change tends to come in fits and starts, often marginal, benefiting only some.

A recent meta-analysis (Rivas, Ramsay, Sadowski, Davidson, Dunne, Eldridge, Hegardy, Taft & Feder, 2015), for example, examined the efficacy of advocacy efforts for women victims of intimate partner violence (IPV). In the 13 studies for over 1,200 abused women, evidence indicated that although some women enjoyed a short-term quality-of-life benefit from advocacy interventions, there was no long-term reduction in the likelihood of future abuse resulting from the advocacy programs.

The National Institute of Justice Crime Solutions webpage is a tool for presenting best practices for scholars, practitioners and policymakers, and studies like Rivas et al.'s project are presented there in terms of what the findings indicate regarding policies and programs. The website presents findings in clear terms: evidence for outcomes from studies is rated using a careful process. Because no significant change occurred for the subjects concerning the likelihood of future abuse, the Rivas et al. study was identified as being "ineffective." Indeed, the researchers in their review of the 13 studies did not find a statistically significant decrease in future abuse, but it did find that there were benefits to some of the women served. It also noted that many of the women were still in their abusive domestic settings at the end of the follow-up period. It would appear to strain credulity to argue that advocacy interventions for women victims of IPV had no appreciable effect. The implication is that advocacy efforts are simply not worth the investment. It seems clear that kind of reasoning includes a preordained institutional bias when evaluating the full ramifications and outcomes of such a study.

Justice is not about the perfection of service. How could it ever be after all? Perfection is not a thing we should seek as humans. Accountability with taxpayer resources matters, to be sure, but it is unproductive to seek to mechanize, routinize or objectivize justice practices through a narrow, self-serving lens. Regardless of how noble justice practitioners may be or how well intentioned, justice defined and confined in terms of objective outcomes, cost–benefit ratios or "best practices" is doomed to mediocrity if a more holistic and inclusive analysis and evaluation is not part of the process.

It would seem clear at this point from all that has come before, that justice and therefore heroism, is much more about honoring our connectedness. Hearing and responding to the voice of the injured other as Simone Weil directs us to do, and responding to the call to enlarge the capacity of our justice system as well as our collective hearts, is as or more important than some kind of objectified, myopic focus on cost–benefit outcomes. Need is not constrained by cost–benefit curves. Neither is justice. Neither are heroes. Neither are heroic leaders.

Heroes are authors of justice in small and big ways Heroism is the process of rendering justice real. Heroes bring justice into being like potters working in clay or painters with pigment on canvas render life-affirming art, or authors shaping narratives in classic works of fiction and nonfiction. We might even go so far as to say that justice is yet another life-affirming art.

The raw materials of that art are humans and their brokenness; the end product is healing, restoration and rehabilitation. In fact, there is just such an art. Kintsugi is the Japanese craft of taking broken pottery and remaking it with gold foil or gold-tinted glue. Kintsugi roughly translates to "repaired with gold." The analogy is a direct one: humans are the pottery, the craftsperson is the hero, the gold foil is heroism and the repaired vessel represents justice in its fullest sense, done. Prisons are full of people who have broken others and themselves through their criminal acts. Correctional officers, counselors, prison superintendents and a host of other prison workers, including volunteers, are each a potential craftsperson. While not all offenders will embrace change nor all corrections professionals will commit to repairing the damage given and received, some will. Some will weave the golden thread of hope and responsibility in creative and incremental ways toward realizing what was lost can become found.

Concluding Remarks

Social science researchers concern themselves with a thing they call self-selection bias. Self-selection bias describes a kind of distortion of research findings that comes from allowing participants to choose themselves for inclusion in a study. If only the high school basketball teams volunteered to show up for the class picture, one might be forgiven for thinking that the school was full of tall folks. Precise descriptions of human phenomena are harder when the thing we seek to understand is exaggerated or hidden. Our examination of heroism here, were it a research project, might be said to suffer from a self-selection-by-proxy bias; "subjects" tell us about significant figures – ordinary heroes – in their lives who did heroic things, who were their heroes. If we wanted a social scientific understanding of heroism, we would want a comparison group, perhaps, of "subjects" to tell us about non-heroes or even "anti-heroes" – folks who might lack other heroic qualities, but who nevertheless rose to the occasion, or just to *an* occasion. This, of course, is not such a project. And it is in no way certain that such a project would produce any greater wisdom and, indeed, might have not included some valuable insights.

The choices that made this work possible, meaning the actions of the ordinary heroes described and illuminated throughout the chapters by students who were the recipients of their encouragement and compassion, offer a kind of experiential virtue that reminds us what the best of humanity looks like and a north star for the rest to try to follow.

What remains now is for you to draw inspiration from these examples, these everyday ordinary heroes of students like yourself, along with the heroes in your own life. Know thyself. Serve from love. Attend to your choices, but forgive when you fail, then learn and try again. Honor what is meaningful: human nurturing and flourishing is our duty. Let no one tell you otherwise: nurturance is wisdom and service is joy. We cannot tell you that every day will be a good one. Some of you will face critical incidents where your lives and the lives of others hang in the balance. Treat yourself kindly but commit yourself fully to the needs you encounter. And when you get lost, know that there are others along the way that will help you, if you have the courage to ask them for directions.

Here at the end, then, it becomes clear: heroes might do difficult things. Sometimes they succeed. Sometimes they fail. They might rush into burning buildings or stand up to bullies. Heroes also sit with you while you do your algebra homework. Heroes may hand-stitch a costume for you for Halloween, even after a long day of hard work. Heroism is about understanding the need of another and serving that need to the greatest of one's ability without thought of return or condition on service. Here at the end it is clear: heroism is nothing more and nothing less than love and our best intentions put into action.

BOX 10.1 LEADERSHIP NOTES

Most of us would like to imagine ourselves doing something heroic in a moment of crisis, like standing up to a bully who is harassing a child, rescuing someone from the path of a speeding car, or saving the day in one way or another. Does our imagination focus more on the moment when self-sacrifice is required – when the outcome is not certain, or more on the accolades received "after" we have saved the day?

The leader whose moral compass is clear and intact is less concerned with the super-hero ensconced in an overactive imagination described above, than in facing an uncertain outcome with all the courage one can muster, to serve those they lead in a time of need. Such a leader's identity is more grounded in being an ordinary hero where the ends do not justify the means. Wholistic concerns are not lost in the meeting of specific goals and needs. Extraordinary purpose, meaning and satisfaction are more likely to result from a personal commitment to servant-leadership than from the grand designs and rhetoric of a pseudo-leader who places a higher priority on being served than on serving others.

Questions

1   From the cases of "ordinary heroes" we have examined, what personal characteristics do you feel exemplify how a hero lives her or his life day to day?
2   What are some of the ethical and moral principles that you would use to describe an effective leader?
3   We end with a final question: What do you want your portrait to be composed of? What do you want your legacy to be?

References

Cummiskey, D. (1990). Kantian consequentialism. *Ethics 100*, 3, 586–615.

DeValve, M. (2015). *A different justice: Love and the future of criminal justice practice in America*. Durham, NC: Carolina Academic Press.

Rivas, C., Ramsay, J., Sadowsky, L., Davidson, L., Dunne, D., Eldridge, S., Hegarty, K., Taft A., & Feder, G. (2015). Advocacy interventions to reduce or eliminate violence and promote the physical and psychological well-being of women who experience intimate partner abuse. *Cochrane Database of Systematic Reviews 3*, 12. DOI: 10.1002/14651858.CD005043. Also referenced from National Institute of Justice Crime Solutions. Accessed May 1, 2020, 9:07pm from https://www.crimesolutions.gov/PracticeDetails.aspx?ID=55

INDEX

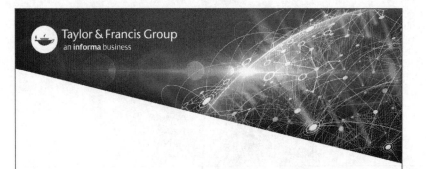